In the Midst of Life

IN THE MIDST OF LIFE

A Hospice Volunteer's Story

CHARLES ROSE

NewSouth Books
Montgomery | Louisville

NewSouth Books
P.O. Box 1588
Montgomery, AL 36102

Copyright © 2007 by Charles Rose
All rights reserved under International and Pan-American Copyright
Conventions. Published in the United States by NewSouth Books, a
division of NewSouth, Inc., Montgomery, Alabama.

Library of Congress Cataloging-in-Publication Data

ISBN 1-60306-020-0

Design by Randall Williams
Printed in the United States of America

For Natalyn

and for my children,
Charles Jr., Mary Elizabeth,
Kenneth, and Sara Josephine

CONTENTS

Preface

I N WRITING THIS BOOK, I realized that the people I came in contact with were turning into faceted and shaped characters, as if they were in a work of fiction. The whole truth about the people in this book can never be known. What I have tried to convey is the impression these people made on me. I have changed the names of patients, caregivers, and others, and, to some extent, I have rearranged and combined certain aspects of the material to heighten narrative immediacy. Yes, this is a narrative, and, as the book will show, something happens to the narrator. More important, I hope something will happen to the reader, that the reader will gain some insight into the actualities of terminal illness and come to appreciate the value of Hospice and other palliative home care organizations.

I

Getting Started

ARLY IN SEPTEMBER 1997, I was sitting in a back booth in Burger King. Putting aside *The Auburn Bulletin*, the weekly local newspaper in Auburn, Alabama, I looked out the window to my left, relieved to see a troop of black high school kids boarding a school bus. Some had taken their drink cups with them, almost all wore Nike or Reebok footwear. A few minutes before they poured into Burger King, I was removing a Whopper Junior with cheese from my tray, a cup of discounted seniors' decaf, water at ten cents a cup. The cacophonous chatter of teen boys and girls deluging the frazzled countermen, how many times had I tuned that out? It didn't stop me from reading *The Bulletin*. I figured I'd take my time, browse through both sections, not just the sports section, anything to ward off kids swarming over the ice and drink dispensers, toting trays to booths, munching Whoppers, Double Cheeseburgers, chunky French fries.

I had an in-progress short story spread out to my left, a cellophane bag of Butterscotch Buttons for the energy surge I used to get from smoking cigarettes, several roller ball pens, a white legal pad. Soon I'd pick up one of those pens, scan the paper, its formidable blankness, wait for words to assemble in my mind, images to crystallize. This had become a daily task, five or six days a week (I had retired from teaching in the English Department at Auburn University in 1994). I wrote in longhand for two to three hours at Burger King, in the same back booth if possible, and did polishing and editing on a Mac Performa at home. Once I got started, the process usually took care of itself, but getting started, that took several Buttons and a continued perusal of *The Bulletin.*

The local goings-on, rendered in an amiably free and easy writing style, were mildly entertaining. I skipped the sports editor's column, "The art of proper heckling," and, on the editorial page, "God is a very present help in trouble." Another column on the editorial page got my attention. "Chaos theory—butterflies effect weather, storms; on the home front too." Shouldn't that be *affect,* I wondered. But as I read on I realized the column wasn't about butterflies thinning out blizzards, but the butterfly effect on the weather, *i.e.,* the enormous impact of a slight meteorological disturbance. The chaos-butterfly theory's formulator, Edward Lorenz, had posed this earth-shaking question: "Could the delicate motion of a butterfly's wings in the Amazon cause a tornado over Texas?" I stopped to ponder this, gazing out to my left, through the long and reassuringly solid glass windows separating my ontological reality from that of the parking lot outside, taking note of the Winnebago with the flat front tire still parked there, a casualty, I used to speculate, of last year's football season, left here far from the stadium by some embittered Auburn Tiger fan over a loss he couldn't come to terms with. "If a tree falls in the forest, Europe will be the less for it," John Donne had written, and Hamlet, foreseeing his own demise, saw "a special Providence in the fall of a sparrow." Now Edward Lorenz was saying interdependence is at work in the weather.

Nothing moved out there in the early September heat, nor were any butterflies around to cool things off. So I went on browsing through Section A until I reached triple columns along the right side of the page, headlined COMMUNITY CALENDAR. The usual items were there. "A meeting for parents of Auburn High ninth through eleventh grade students," "A Lee-Scott Academy 'Moms in Touch' meeting," "Auburn Mommy and me . . . Dads welcome too!, a free parent support-child play group will meet weekly to promote positive parenting and to provide interaction among children." "Auburn University SGA will hold a blood drive from 9 A.M. to 5 P.M. in the Haley Center Basement." I used to teach in Haley Center, a nine-story building towering over the campus, and often passed, without ever volunteering myself, the curtained-off area for giving blood after having a snack in the basement cafeteria.

Under the subheading "Join Project Uplift" I read that caring volunteers were needed to work with Lee County children. This I had thought about doing, but so far I hadn't signed on. Now that I had retired from teaching, I had the time to perform some kind of social service. My wife, Natalyn, and I had talked about my joining the local literacy program, but procrastination had prevailed. I glanced under Outreach Program, smiled at a "workshop, "Storytelling: Finding Your Voice," to be held at Pebble Hill, an old Southern mansion recently refurbished for literary readings and coffee klatches. No, not for me, I said to myself. Then I came on the subheading "Become a Hospice Volunteer." "Call 887-4546 for information on volunteer training sessions in October." My hand lingered on a Butterscotch Button.

I knew somebody who was in Hospice, Marnie Hudson. She was a massage therapist I went to once a month. I was one of her clients, along with many Auburn friends. To get to Marnie's place one had to drive northwest on U.S. 280 to Waverly, a hamlet replete with antique stores and unreconstructed hippies, then drive another five miles through the boondocks, negotiating ruts and potholes. She had told me once she did massages for the terminally ill. The next time I went out there, I said to myself, why not ask her to tell me more about what working for Hospice was all about?

A week or ten days later, I was drinking the glass of cool well water Marnie has waiting for her clients when they come out of the massage room. When I finished the water, I wrote out a check for thirty-five dollars and set up my next appointment. An attractive woman in her early forties, she sat opposite me at her desk, her appointment book laid out in front of her. She wrote the date and time on the back of an appointment card, and, as usual, handed it over to me.

I remembered what she had told me earlier that afternoon. She had been giving massage therapy to her latest Hospice patient, an older woman she had become attached to. "She's in a bad way, I'm thinking. I don't expect her to last much longer." Marnie's voice showed concern, her blue-green eyes hazing over. Now that I was about to leave (another client would be showing up soon), I knew I had to ask what doing Hospice meant to her.

She told me she felt her connection with Hospice was life-enhancing. Being with the terminally ill took her out of herself. And she knew she was doing something worthwhile, that the patients she saw responded to her, that in some mysterious way she could connect with them. She didn't show an undue fascination with death and dying, characteristic of so many good folks in these parts. She talked about her patients the way she'd talk about transplanting canna lilies or mowing the tall grass in her big backyard. Listening to her, I was rapidly becoming persuaded that serving as a Hospice volunteer was something I might really do, so I asked Marnie how one got started. She was pleased that I was interested. She told me where the Hospice offices were, in the fitness center building on Dean Road, not that far from where I lived. First I'd have to go to training sessions, which were scheduled for late October. I didn't tell Marnie I already knew about the training sessions. I did say I might need some time to make a decision.

Marnie gave me a look of mild disparagement. "Well, just be sure you don't wait too long. If you don't sign on and take the training, you'll have to wait another year to get started. You wouldn't want to do that, would you? That would look like procrastination to me."

"No, I wouldn't want to do that," I replied, noting the woodcut above her desk, depicting a gaunt St. Francis feeding some very scrawny birds. "Next year would be way too late."

DRIVING BACK ON LEE COUNTY 28, I had to slow down for stretches of washboard road. I was crawling along in second gear, the red clover thick on each side of the road. I'd pick up speed, have to slow down again. Speeding up, having to slow down again, it got me thinking about where I was at this point in my life.

I had retired from teaching at Auburn University, as an Associate Professor Emeritus, having put in thirty-four years in the English Department. I would never have to grade another freshman theme or student term paper. I could read a book without having to take notes, prepare a syllabus, or wade through criticism. I'd kept to a writing schedule, putting in four or five hours a day, for five days a week. I had had several stories accepted; one had even been nominated for The Pushcart Prize by *The Chattahoochee Review*. I had a novel underway. I had other activities—playing blues and standards on the piano, drawing, coloring, and mounting Napoleonic soldiers, uniforms authentic, in various postures of hostility and heroism. I continued to play tennis, winning a set now and then, in spite of increasingly painful surges of tendonitis after a match.

My wife Natalyn and I had our customary ways. A widely exhibited artist, Natalyn did her work in the garage studio in the mornings. I'd sleep in, get up, potter around the house, play the piano, pay some bills. Early in the afternoon I went off to write at Burger King. I'd read through *The Auburn Bulletin*, then write longhand for two or three hours. Then, returning to 305 Bowden Drive, I'd sit down at the computer, rewrite for two hours or so. Natalyn and I would have two or three drinks. After a late dinner we watched television, or a movie on video or did crossword puzzles. Still later, we did our reading. During those times when Natalyn was busy getting ready for an exhibition, I did the dishes, kept the kitchen cleaned up.

On holidays and occasionally during the year, I saw my children, Charles and Mary, Kenneth and Josephine, in their thirties now, married, with children of their own. Divorce had left its imprint on them. Yet we were still close. The bad times, what had led to divorces, the turbulence and suffering that had ensued, seemed a long way in the past.

I crossed a narrow bridge over the railroad about five miles away from Waverly. The road leveled out, the ruts giving way to tar-speckled asphalt. For a moment, I felt I was in the middle of nowhere, on my way from one place to another without knowing why. It came over me—what was I doing for others, apart from those who were close to me? I wasn't likely to turn a beggar away, but did that make me a good Samaritan?

In the past, my support of worthy causes hadn't been impressive. I hadn't participated in the civil rights movement, although as a fledgling assistant professor at Auburn I had supported it at a distance, in the classroom, not out in the streets. I had opposed the Viet Nam war from my cozy, professorial armchair, reading about all the protesting with a comforting bourbon and water close at hand. At the time there was little student and faculty protest over Viet Nam at Auburn University. In the late sixties, I did sign a bail bond mortgaging my home to enable two bedraggled seventeen-year-old girls up on a possession charge to gain release from the ruck and filth of the Opelika jail. Fortunately, the girls showed up for their trial, and I wasn't out anything.

The sun faded behind banks of dense cumuli as I drove on, making little progress it seemed. I got stuck behind a log truck and had to slow down again, hanging far enough away from the red flag so I could swerve if the slanted-down tree trunks came unwedged. Playing it safe even now, I continued to ask myself why I needed to be doing Hospice. Something came to me from Carson McCullers, what twelve-year-old Frankie Addams realizes in *The Member of the Wedding*—she's searching for the "we of me." Frankie thinks she will fulfill herself by honeymooning with her brother and her brother's bride. But she finally realizes that it is her connection with the black housekeeper, Berenice, and her cousin, John Henry, that matters. What they shared during that long summer in the Addams kitchen is beginning to shape her "we of me." Out of context, the line was close to an existential catchword, but now, in the light of what I was considering, it took on a renewed significance.

I realized I hadn't been around the terminally ill, and didn't know how I'd handle it. A memory from childhood seized hold of me—my Aunt Ethel suffering from cancer. She'd been sealed up in an upstairs room in my grandmother's house. When my brother and I came to visit, we weren't taken upstairs to see Aunt Ethel. But one night, for some reason, we were upstairs. Her bedroom door was open, and we saw her. Her jaw was swollen the size of a grapefruit, and we could almost feel her throbbing anguish. She looked shapeless in her narrow bed, her narrow room, with nothing to cling to but the radio muttering into her ears.

Other memories, my father dying suddenly, at age sixty-six,

of gangrene poisoning from acute phlebitis. I was in Auburn six hundred miles away from my hometown of Kokomo, Indiana, not at my father's bedside. My mother lived on to age eighty-seven. I'd seen my mother a week before she died, visited at her duplex on North Taylor Street. She seemed in good health at the time. She still had her special martini at night, gin laced with olive juice, a touch of vermouth, prepared meat loaf and macaroni and cheese for me, sliced tomatoes dappled with mayonnaise, which we ate at the kitchen table. She still watched Johnny Carson and Indiana University basketball games. She did complain of diarrhea. She'd been having the runs for weeks now. She told me she'd been taking Pepto-Bismol, but it hadn't helped much.

Before I left to go back to Auburn, I talked my mother into checking into the hospital. She wouldn't go as long as I was there, but not long after I left she did. She called me the night she got there, and left her number, and I called her back. We talked for nearly an hour. She seemed in good spirits, and said she was so glad she was there. Two nights later her neighbor telephoned me from the hospital. My mother was going fast, could I get up there? Perhaps I could have gotten a last-minute flight out of Atlanta or Birmingham, but I didn't, I stayed where I was. My mother died later that night. The cause of death was said to be heart failure. We never found out what it really was. Margaret Johnson, her neighbor, who truly cared for her, was with her when she died. She was a good churchgoing Methodist, and she told my mother Jesus would take her soon. I wouldn't have been able to do that.

I had been able to be at my daughter Sara Josephine's side while she went through four successive operations for an abscessed colon, resulting from a flare-up in her Crohn's disease. Josephine was nineteen, a sophomore at the University of the South, on two scholarships, an outstanding student. I spent the weekends (I was teaching during the week) in Josephine's hospital room, at Crawford Long Hospital, in Atlanta. I sat beside Josephine throughout the day and most of the night, sleeping fitfully on an improvised cot in the small hours of the morning, my vigil relieved by breakfast and dinner break, at an upscale restaurant across the street from the hospital. At times, I tried to distance myself by reading one of the novels I was teaching in modern British lit, Margaret Drabble's *The Ice Age*, but that didn't help for very long at a time. The second operation was the worst. Locked in behind the log truck, I remembered holding Josephine's hand when the pain was bad, praying for her to get through it.

I had to slow down while the log truck crossed a narrow plank bridge over a railroad cut, not far from Waverly. Once the truck was over and on down the road, I rattled over the bridge myself. Sunbeams sliced through banks of cumuli, gilding bungalows set back from the road, doublewide trailers, satellite dishes, a presumptuous placard in a lonely front yard announcing V-BALL PLAYED HERE, CALL 826-1812, its volleyball net stretched tight. On my right, set back from the road, a brick house with a portico and columns, big shade trees, a driveway and stables. Then I was driving through the north fringe of Waverly, turning left onto U.S. 280. The log truck took a turn to the right, toward Alexander City. I left my memories of sickness and death behind, but my "we of me," why not try bringing it out? Picking up speed on the highway, I told myself I had made up my mind.

A WEEK LATER I SUBMITTED an application. At that time located on Dean Road, Hospice of EAMC (East Alabama Medical Center) occupied a jutting wing of Auburn Fitness, another bodybuilding, pumping-iron establishment. The swimming pool glittered unenticingly, a turquoise rectangle set in bleak concrete. I moved on out of the parking lot toward the glass doors, spirea bushes rustling on either side as I pushed the doors open and entered the reception room. A mousy young woman in a pale pink blouse gave me an application, and I took a seat and filled it out. The condolence cards thumbtacked to bulletin boards, the artificial flowers—that would take some getting used to. Being outside again was a relief. But I'd taken the first step. The next day I got a call from the volunteers coordinator, Bill Wanamaker. We arranged for an interview on Monday morning of the following week.

The reception room hadn't changed when I got back. All it needed was a solicitous undertaker's assistant to turn it into a funeral home. But when Bill Wanamaker came striding in, I felt better. He pulled a chair up and sat, turning my way to make his presence felt. He was a good-sized man with a tufted gray beard and prematurely gray hair. He wore an open-collared, candy-striped shirt and navy blue gabardine slacks with a crease. He held a clipboard with my application, which was about all that was official or institutional in this, my first interview with him.

Bill didn't take long to let me know we'd met before. "You may not remember me, Dr. Rose, but I had European novel with you once." He went on to say something about the books we'd read—Dostoyevsky, Kafka, Mann, Camus, how important they had been for him. He must have done some hard thinking before he'd taken this job. He leaned forward, his fingertips touching, as he spoke, seriously yet informally, filling me in on what Hospice was all about. He told me Hospice provides care at the home for terminally ill patients and their families. It provides benefits that aren't available in hospitals, nursing homes, and other institutional settings. It serves the family as a unit and is sensitive to special needs. As a volunteer, I would be part of a team that included a physician, a nurse, a clergyman, a social worker, homecare aides, and physical and occupational therapists. Part of a team, yes, but when it comes down to the most important thing, being there for the patient and his family, the volunteer is indispensable.

Bill paused to see how I was responding. A bit put off, I told Bill I liked what the Hospice was doing but I wasn't sure being a volunteer was for me.

Bill gave his beard a tug, as if he were the teacher now and he was pondering what to say next to a not very responsive student. "That's understandable, Dr. Rose. If you do this you'll be getting to know people you might not have been in contact with. And although you might not think so now, you're going to become attached to these people."

I said I understood that might happen, that was just it. "Getting close to someone who is dying, that's something I may not be cut out for. It's too easy for me to distance myself."

Bill eased his big shoulders against the back of the chair. "I just want you to understand you can be of service." I saw the receptionist look up uneasily from her desk. "Not only that, we're a little short of men your age right now. When I say you could be of service, I'm thinking most men who are terminal would rather have another guy around. An older man, someone about the same age."

I hadn't thought of that, and said so.

"Well, I thought of it when I got your application. That you were someone we could really use. And there are things you could do, like, why not read stories to them, or poetry? I mean you're good at reading aloud; it's something you did as a teacher." Bill let his shoulders relax a little, and quietly recited the last two lines of "The Second Coming." "'And what rough beast his hour come round at last / Slouches toward Bethlehem to be born.' I heard you do that in sophomore lit. In case you don't remember I was there, I was the kid in the back row who never said anything. But believe me I was taking it in."

I had an easy answer for that one, visualizing Bill in the back row, the hangdog look, the sophomoric, unYeatsian slouch of a loner, a searcher. "You were young. Your life was ahead of you then."

"That's right, I was young and eager. And a lot of my life is still ahead of me." Bill stretched out his long legs, pulling the clipboard off his knees. "These people, their lives are behind them. But you don't know what effect you might have on them. If only by being there for them." He was on his feet, standing over me. "Well, think about it. There's really a way for you to fit in. Or you could start out in the office. Get your feet wet, if that's how you want to go. Either way you will have to do the training. I will have to have a commitment from you on that."

I hesitated for a few seconds. Then— "You can sign me up for the training. After that, I'll see."

"Fair enough," Bill said. "See what happens." He shoved the clipboard under one arm and filled me in on what was ahead. The training was set for late October. He'd send me a schedule in September. We shook hands in front of the glass doors, and I was on my way to the parking lot, feeling good about what I was getting involved in.

Midway in the first training session, somewhere around 7 p.m., five women and three men, including myself, were sitting on either side of a long table, about to view our first video, entitled "Making Each Day Count." Two middle-aged conventional Southern white women, one middle-aged conventional black woman, one shy young woman with acne, and a skittish white Auburn University coed. There were two male AU students sitting side-by-side, well-dressed, well-groomed, muscled bodybuilders with very dedicated expressions on their faces. Kevin Johnson, the white male, had worked in the office; the black male, Bill Doak, had just come on board. They didn't seem to know quite what to make of me, a shaggy-haired, gray-mustached ex-prof, and I was careful to keep my distance from them.

A paper plate from the snack bar sat in front of me, potato chips, scattered mixed nuts, a few pretzels, and a paper cup half full of Sprite going flat. I nibbled on nuts while we waited to get started. For awhile, Bill Wanamaker had one eye on the door, hoping for some late arrival. He finally looked at his watch, and we got started. Bill began by thanking us for coming, and went on to describe the opportunity ahead of us. He passed out Hospice folders containing a schedule, the do's and don'ts involved in a volunteer's conduct, Hospice Initial Database sheets, Hospice Volunteer Direct Patient Care Family Activity sheets to be filled out after each visit, and a wealth of material on the dying process and the grieving process. Then it was time for us to watch the video. Bill dimmed the fluorescent lights.

For me, the video was a little overdone. I watched saintly volunteers ministering to sweet-tempered patients. The sound track was unnecessarily rhapsodical. Finally, it was over. Bill switched on the lights.

On the way home that night, I realized that, even though "Making Each Day Count" might to some extent falsify actuality, my response was little more than a distancing process, a way of getting away from why I was there. On the whole, the training sessions were stimulating and informative, if a little drawn out. We had four hours a night to cover what might have been covered in three. One thing that stretched out the sessions was filling out a questionnaire for each training aspect, a way of evaluating the presentation. We sat around the table for fifteen minutes or so checking boxes—Excellent, Very Good, Good, Below Average, Poor. I think I checked Excellent for everybody.

On the night of our second session Bill went over what was in each of our folders, covering everything I might need to know. One thing he stressed was confidentiality, and another was exactitude in the reports we were required to turn in, concerning time spent, mileage, kinds of service performed (run errands, help pay bills, provide cassette tapes for listening, etc.). On the third night, the bereavement director, Annie Nelson, took us through Elizabeth Kubler-Ross's five stages of bereavement: denial, anger, bargaining, depression, acceptance. Annie also suggested things we might do, from going to visitations, attending funerals, following up with visits to the bereaved in which we were to encourage reminiscence and urge other therapeutic measures when appropriate. On the fourth night, a nurse from East Alabama Medical Center, a highly professional and knowledgeable middle-aged black woman who struck me as having seen it all, explained pain relief, one of Hospice's chief objectives. She emphasized the need to alleviate pain, no matter what. Acute pain seldom lasted long, and there were usually ways to deal with it. I learned that a patient can be given up to one thousand milligrams of morphine a day, that relief for chronic pain can be partially achieved through guided imagery and massage therapy. The nurse went on to describe the dying process: the patient becomes weaker, spends more time in bed, is unable to move around, exhibits decreased appetite. There is an increase in breathing problems, a decline in body temperature, fluid collecting in the back of the throat, finally, the well-known death rattle. On that same night the Hospice chaplain described the emotional experience, what was going on with the dying. He said they saw themselves living their metaphors, going on a journey, crossing a river, laying down a burden.

After the training was over, I put off getting started. I had an excuse for procrastination. Before I could be assigned a patient, it was necessary for me to take a tuberculosis test. If the test came out positive, I would have to get an X-ray at the county health clinic. If negative, I could go ahead and get started. The problem here, enabling me to postpone taking the test, concerned my wife

Natalyn's hospitalization a year ago. She'd been given a TB test in the hospital, and it had turned out positive. So there was a possibility she might be a carrier. If so, I might be a carrier myself. Since I could only take the test once a year, I felt that Natalyn should have the X-ray first. If she was not a carrier I could take the test with some confidence that it would turn out right, thereby sparing me a trip, and a long wait, at the clinic.

Natalyn put off the X-ray until December. As it turned out, the X-ray showed she was not a carrier, so I was free to take the test myself, which I did early in January. It amounted to two inoculations of a weakened strain of the virus, taken at intervals two weeks apart. The results were good; I was negative.

By February, I was aware that the TB test had become a meticulously elaborate avoidance mechanism. Bill couldn't match me up with the right person for another month. In late March he did have someone, a cancer patient, Brian Stapler. Brian Stapler's family owned a restaurant outside Auburn, on the Opelika Road this side of the Mall. Early in April Bill telephoned to tell me that Brian Stapler's wife had made other arrangements. In May, Bill called me again. He had a black man, Alonzo Simmons, whose prostrate cancer had metastasized. We could go to his place early next week.

2

Women on the Porch

L ONNIE SIMMONS HAS BEEN in a coma for weeks, his
sister, Mary Wagner tells me. His eyes are closed, his lips
are parted, he's unable to breathe without an oxygen machine. His prostate cancer has metastasized; he hasn't got long to
live. He's lying in a hospital bed, his wristwatch looped around
one of the legs of the bed, in a house he does not own but has
lived in for the last thirty years. The bed is parallel to the front
window. If Lonnie would open his eyes, turn his head a little, he
would be able to see the photograph of a woman, on the television
set, the woman he lived with for years. Her image, all he has left
of her, may still be with him.

From the Hospice Initial Data Sheet:

Description of Present Status

KPS 40%, vis stable B/P 11074 P86R20

Awake, alert, oriented. 54 year old black male

metastatic prostate: cancer bone metes. c./o.

severe pain, now controlled c oxcartin 40 mg,

use as Lartab PRN. No bowel movement since

last week. Family need assistance, unable to do

any activities at present, unable to stand.

Lonnie is seventy-six, not fifty-four. And he isn't awake, he isn't alert.

THE FIRST TIME I saw them they were sitting out on the front porch of the house Lonnie rented on Hager Place, a side street off Jeter Avenue on the east side of Opelika. Mary Wagner was Lonnie's sister, Jo-Anne Simmons was his daughter.

Bill parked in front of the house. We got out of the car. I watched Bill stride up the walk ahead of me. In his candy-striped shirt, beltless light gray slacks, tan loafers, Bill seemed out of place here; yet his connection to Hospice made a difference. I could tell Bill was accepted here. But I was a stranger. The women sitting out on the front porch viewed me with uncertainty and mistrust. Right away, I noticed Jo-Anne's tan sunglasses with tiger-striped rims.

We didn't go into the house right away. Bill introduced me, adding that I used to be a professor at Auburn University. Mary asked me what I taught, and I told her English composition and literature, adding that I had taught for thirty-four years but was currently enjoying my retirement. We stayed on the porch in the mild May heat while Mary finished her cigarette. "How's Lonnie doing?" Bill asked Mary, and she told him, in a matter-of-fact-way, that Lonnie was quiet today. Yesterday afternoon he had pitched a fit. She had had to hold him down until the nurse arrived. The nurse had said Lonnie needed more morphine. The nurse couldn't give the morphine to Lonnie by mouth, so she had to insert it into his rectum.

Mary exhibited a knowing air I was to encounter again. By filling me in on Ronnie's condition she was able to distance herself from Ronnie's suffering.

"He can hear you but he can't talk," she said, for she needed to believe Lonnie knew she was there.

I drifted in close to the oxygen machine, which was bubbling with every racking breath Lonnie took. Bill wedged himself between the hospital bed and the air-conditioner in the window. A gray sheet that hung from a curtain rod over the front window stirred. Had the sheet been there while Lonnie was healthy or had Mary put it up after he took sick? From where I was standing, Lonnie's face was turned away. My eyes on a man in a coma, I waited for something to happen. Finally, Bill came out with, "Lonnie, this is your Hospice volunteer," his voice professional, reassuring. Staring at the back of Lonnie's head, I blurted out, "I'm pleased to meet you, Lonnie."

Bill gave me a look that made me realize Lonnie didn't know who was talking to him. I moved on around the head of the bed and sidled past Bill to the air-conditioner. Now I was standing over Lonnie, looking down at his face, the high forehead, the grizzled hair, the parted lips, the lowered eyelids. I was less than three feet away from him. I said, "Lonnie, I'm Charlie. Charlie Rose. I'm your Hospice volunteer." I couldn't detect a response. I said to him, I'd be back next week, Tuesday morning. Yes, I would see him then, I said firmly, as if I were announcing some big event in his life.

Bill signaled to me, we shouldn't say much longer. Then I was leaving the churning oxygen machine behind, the plastic bag hanging at the foot of the bed holding Lonnie's urine, his feces. I was ready to go, and I sensed Bill was too. Nonetheless, our leave-taking was leisurely. We made small talk on the front porch. It wouldn't do for us to run off right away; Mary and Jo-Anne realized that too. Sunlight glittered in the pecan tree, a slight breeze shuffling the leaves.

On the way back to Auburn, we drove through Opelika, staying on Highway 29. Bill Wanamaker wasn't in any hurry to get back, so we drove through town, then on past East Alabama Medical

Center, the Wal-Mart shopping plaza, the multiplex theater, the Mall. Bill told me stories he'd heard from his grandmother, about what it was like in Opelika during the Second World War. There used to be prostitutes walking the streets, for Opelika had been a stopover for outbound troops from Fort Benning. A German POW camp had been in Opelika, out south on U.S. 169, where Uniroyal is located now. The POW's did yard work for people in town. When the war was over, Bill informed me, some of them settled in the South.

Bill dropped me off at the new Hospice building. Once I was in my car, it overwhelmed me, what I'd experienced that morning. The leaves seemed greener, the sun felt good. I had been in the presence of immanent, inescapable death. What to do? Why do anything? Or is there some way one can amend one's life? An image of African-American women on a front porch, a dying man's face in drugged acquiescence. I felt tears start. Lonnie was dying. For a moment or two, familiar sights, Dean Road, Kroger's, Glendean Drugs, seemed mysteriously sentient.

Four days later, I was approaching Mary Wagner, sitting out on her front porch, by herself this time. I was on my own. Bill Wanamaker wouldn't be propping me up today. I made a mistake right off the bat. I got her name wrong; I confused her with Jo-Anne Simmons. I called Mary Wagner, Jo-Anne. Mary looked as if she'd been lightly slapped, yet she managed to keep a smile on her face. "No, I'm Mary," she said, and I remembered Jo-Anne's tigerish sunglasses. I blurted out something, oh sorry. Next time I'll get it right.

Mary was wearing the same matching dark blue blouse and skirt. The nurse was with Lonnie at the time, so we sat outside on the porch for awhile. I didn't really want Mary to leave, even though that was what I was there for, to give her a little respite. It was getting on toward lunch time, and so I asked Mary if she wanted to go somewhere. She might want to get some lunch or pick up something in a supermarket.

Mary said to me, without appearing to think about it, "I'd rather stay here. I'd just like to be with somebody. We could just talk if you don't mind."

"I don't mind. I'd like that too."

A little while before the nurse came out, Jo-Anne sauntered over from across the street. Both women went inside the house to confer with the nurse. After the nurse left, Jo-Anne said she wanted to sit out on the porch with Mary, and I said I would sit with Lonnie awhile. Mary asked me if I wanted something to drink. I said I'd have a Diet Coke.

"I can give you a Diet Pepsi," Mary said.

"That's fine. I'll have that."

I followed Mary inside. Lonnie was still lying on the hospital bed. Mary told him the man from Hospice was here, here to see you, Lonnie. There was an armchair near the kitchen; Mary motioned for me to sit down in it. Instead I went to Lonnie and told him who I was and why I was here. He didn't respond; he just lay there. His eyes were closed, he was breathing hard.

"He may not show it but he can hear you," Mary said, handing me a cold can of Diet Pepsi. "You sure you want to sit with him?"

"I'll sit with him. You go have your cigarette." Without glancing at Lonnie, Mary went out to join Jo-Anne on the porch.

I was alone with Lonnie. For a little while, the floor fan's whicker, the ceiling fan's wobbly counterpoint had a soothing effect on me. That and the oxygen machine's uninterrupted bubbling helped to keep me from thinking about the man in the bed. I concentrated on Lonnie's breathing. I thought of it graphed in repeated waves. A sliding ascent, a swift descent. HAAA-AAHHFFT. Then HAUGHT and two short beats. A

glissando up—HAAAAAHHFFT. Sharp drop down. HAUGHT
TWO THREE. Gliding dance step AWONNNNNNN and
ONETWOTHREE.

About forty minutes, the minute hand creeping on my wristwatch, went by. Then Mary came back inside. After poking her
head inside the door to say good-bye to us, Jo-Anne returned to
her house across the street. I felt better now that Mary was here.
She went on into the kitchen and came back with a kitchen chair.
She sat down across from me, by the front door, a little behind
Lonnie. His toes were pointed away from us, his reversed head im-
mobile. I'd offered Mary the armchair without actually getting up.
No thank you, she said, she wanted me to have the armchair.

We tried to talk. For awhile, the conversation was pretty
one-sided. Mary did most of the talking. As she had said when I
arrived, she needed to talk to someone. She told me some things
about Lonnie. For years he'd driven a truck for Pepperell Mill.
Eleven years ago, he'd had his legs crushed. Cotton bales had fallen
out of the back of a truck, had knocked him down, pinned him
against the concrete slab. He'd had the fractured bones broken
again and reset, but he wasn't ever the same afterwards. Lonnie,
Mary confided, was a drinker, and he had a girl friend who had
lived with him these last few years. Mary pointed out the woman's
photograph to me. "That's her sitting on the TV." She said she
herself hadn't been that close to Lonnie, but someone had to be
with him now. It was hard, but she had to do it. "The Lord will
help me get through this" she said, a quiet conviction in her voice.
She couldn't believe the things she had been able to do. But she'd
known the Lord would give her the strength.

I sensed that Mary wanted to say more, so I asked her how long
Lonnie had been ill. Since February, she told me. Lonnie hadn't
told her he had a prostate condition. His hip had been hurting
him, that was in February, a little over three months ago. The pain

had spread to his spine, his ribs. Mary and Jo-Anne had taken him to the cancer center at East Alabama Medical Center. He had had bone surgery there, radiation and chemotherapy throughout February, on into March. Late in March, he was admitted to Hospice, and not long after that Lonnie's neighbor, Herman Hall, had called her. Herman had told her Lonnie couldn't take care of himself, and Herman couldn't be with him all the time. So Mary had moved into Lonnie's house. She had applied to the Veterans Administration Hospital at Tuskegee. It would be months before a bed there would be available. Lonnie couldn't stand up or go to the bathroom. It wasn't long before he couldn't eat. He was too far gone to take an I.V., his veins were too brittle. She fed him liquids out of an eyedropper. Like feeding a baby, she told me.

About that time, Herman Hall came in, a middle-aged, stoop-shouldered black man. Mary went out on the porch to smoke a cigarette. Herman didn't waste time talking to me; he went straight to Lonnie. He looked down at Lonnie, put his hand on Lonnie's emaciated arm and said, "Old friend, how you doin'?" His voice was low pitched, tinctured with sadness. "Hope you get better," Herman said to Lonnie. Turning toward me, he said, "'preciate your stoppin' by." Then he was out the door, on his way.

Mary came back inside and we talked some more. This time we had more to say. I filled her in on my four children, my five grandchildren, leaving out the two divorces, other matters. Then Mary filled me in on her grandchildren. One was going to a trade school, another was in the military. She said she had worked hard to keep her daughter in school. Her daughter was a nurse now. Not all of her children had managed to stay in school. The grandson who was now in trade school, he'd fooled around, dropped out of school, but she thought he was on the right track now.

She went on to tell me she had diabetes. Some years ago her blood sugar was low and for three weekends running she'd lost her sight. The Lord had given her strength to get through it. I said I knew something about diabetes because my father-in-law had had it. He had given himself an insulin shot every night. Yes, I know, Mary said, I've had to do that.

The television set had been on mute throughout our conversation. Mary offered to turn it off; that would be up to her, I said. She said she'd just as soon turn it off. I asked her if she watched a lot of television, and she said that although she had her favorites, there wasn't that much on the television that appealed to her. She did watch "The Oprah Winfrey Show" and "Wheel of Fortune." I asked her whether "Wheel of Fortune" was on now, and she said, no not until evening. Our conversation continued to limp along. What we were saying seemed arbitrary, disconnected, for we were clinging to a conventional wisdom in order to hold off Lonnie's presence.

The paneled half curtains on the window the bed faced, the window that housed the window fan (I realized there were three fans, not two), we had a pair of curtains like them in one of our bedrooms, black and white checked half curtains looped around a curtain rod. They were from Big Lots or Wal-Mart, I didn't recall which. My wife and I had picked them out. Natalyn would buy kitchen items at Big Lots, thick rolls of trash bags, garbage bags, detergents, Saran wrap, Tupperware. Lonnie's curtains might have come from Wal-Mart.

"I have some curtains like yours at my home," I said to Mary. "They have the same pattern as yours."

"Is that right. You know, Lonnie picked these out himself. They really look nice, don't they?"

Another sister, whose name I can't remember, came in a little later. She looked like Mary in the face, but her hair was gray and she had put on fat. She got to talking about her husband. He had Alzheimer's disease, her husband did, and like Lonnie, her husband was on the waiting list at the V.A. Hospital. We talked about Alzheimer's for awhile.

I had a colleague who had gotten Alzheimer's. That was in the mid-seventies. His name was Bernard Goldman. Bernard Goldman was the senior professor in modern lit. He hadn't published a lot, but he was a good man and a fine teacher. I didn't say much about Bernie. What I said was—in the early stages of his disease, Bernie still had coffee with me. He'd walk from his home, almost a mile away from Haley Center, and take the elevator up to the ninth floor, go to the coffee room, and sit with his colleagues. Once, sitting with him in the coffee room, he had said to me, "You know, Charlie, Saul Bellow, he's a fine writer, isn't he?" Bernard Goldman was trying to carry on—but I couldn't really convey that to Mary and her sister. Mary's sister was saying about her husband, "when it rains, he won't come out of his room. He doesn't know where he is half the time. He doesn't know where to go to the bathroom."

At some point in the conversation, a young black woman from down the street dropped in. She was slender, attractive, self-assured. She had been a Hospice nurse herself at one time. Now she was a nurse at East Alabama Medical Center. She told me Hospice did a lot of good things. Her gaze was direct and open. I felt she wouldn't tolerate condescending remarks from a white person so she wouldn't say much to me. But she appreciated my being there.

This pretty woman went to Lonnie and said something to him. I got up out of the armchair when the young woman said she had to be going. We shook hands, in a detached, professional way.

Before I left, I did a drawing of Mary sitting in a ladderback chair, her hands folded, a little smile on her face. I showed the drawing to her. Her eyes lit up, she liked it. She showed it to her sister, and her sister said it looked just like her. Then I got up and went to Lonnie. He was breathing hard. His mouth was open, his hands flopped outside the wrinkled sheet covering him from his chest to his ankles. Suddenly, his belly lurched, heaving the sheet up. Then he was quiet again. I told him I'd be back on Friday. "I'll see you on Friday, Lonnie."

Driving back to Auburn, I took I-85 to Auburn instead of driving through Opelika. I thought of Bernie Goldman, before Alzheimer's hit him. Bernie had been the director of graduate studies in the English literature program. His office was part of a sectioned-off block of departmental offices, at one end of the ninth floor of Haley Center. One afternoon, as I was leaving my own office, plodding down the hall to the elevator—was I hearing things or was that the Benny Goodman Quartet (Clarinet, B. Goodman, Vibraphone, L. Hampton, Piano, T. Wilson, Drums, G. Krupa) swinging lickety split through "Avalon"? Bernie was playing the tape in his office. I went in and there he was—gazing out the window at the football stadium as some of the best jazz you'll ever hear broke through ice floes of academic propriety. Turning to me, Bernie said, "I thought these guys might liven things up around here."

"LONNIE, I'M GOING to give you a little water. It's time for your morphine. It's time for your morphine, Lonnie."

Mary Wagner has already explained to me how it is done, giving Lonnie morphine by mouth. She lays an eye dropper on the tip of his tongue. He has opened his mouth. He won't have to swallow, she tells me, because the liquid is absorbed through a membrane of the tongue. Mary finishes, inserting the eyedropper into a small glass bottle. She sets the bottle down on a table behind the oxygen machine.

I don't ask her how much morphine she has given him. The nurse who talked to us Hospice volunteers at one of our training sessions said you can give a patient up to one thousand milligrams of morphine a day, whatever makes the patient comfortable. The nurse said a lot of physicians don't prescribe enough morphine. Since morphine locks the bowels, she said, you have to give enemas periodically. I wondered whether Mary did that, or did the Hospice nurse who came twice a week?

IT'S FRIDAY, MAY EIGHTH. I'm on my third visit here. Herman Hall drops by. He says he's going out for Kentucky Fried. Mary asks me if Herman can get me some chicken. Selfishly, I think of losing weight; I tell Herman I'll have a doughnut.

'What kind," Herman inquires, "glazed or chocolate?"

"Glazed," I say.

Herman moves a little closer to me. "Could I get you some fried okra?"

"Sure. That's sounds good."

Herman and Mary go off to Kentucky Fried. I'm with Lonnie. I take note of his breathing. A short intake, long exhalation. In five beats—one two three four five. Rising , slowly falling. It isn't long before Herman and Mary are back. Herman hands me two Krispy Kreme glazed doughnuts in a cardboard carton, another carton containing fried okra. Presently, Mary drifts over to my chair. Will I have a piece of chicken? I can't turn her down; besides, I'm hungry. I take a drumstick. Herman follows Mary out to the porch. They'll have their lunch on the porch. Still with Lonnie, I eat the drumstick first—it's still warm—then I peck away at the crisp, chewy, fried okra. Finally, I tackle the doughnuts. Herman Hall must have made an extra stop for the doughnuts; I tell myself—you need to eat both doughnuts.

Later, two black Hospice workers come to change Lonnie's sheets, and bathe him—Melissa, light-skinned, coral blue lipstick liberally applied, and Virginia, her buxom co-worker. After Mary introduces us, I excuse myself, and go out to the front porch. It isn't long before Mary joins me. We sit on the porch a while, not saying much, until Melissa and Virginia are finished.

THIS HAS TO DO with reading the Bible aloud. The night before I was to be with Lonnie, I thought about what I would read to him. I didn't know what his condition would be today. I thought I'd read something from the Old Testament, a self-contained, familiar story, and after reading through Joshua and through much about David and Saul (David, I learned, went off into the woods at one point, like Hamlet, feigning madness), I settled on David and Goliath. 1 Samuel, Chapter 17. Before Mary gave Lonnie the morphine, before she put the eyedropper to his lips, while she was still sitting out on the front porch, smoking a cigarette, chatting with Jo-Anne, I got up from my armchair and went to the hospital bed. I pulled the Bible out of a cloth bag.

On my right, I heard the bubbling oxygen machine. Lonnie's breathing hadn't changed, still the short rise, the long exhalation. I opened the Bible to the place I had marked.

> And David put his hand in his bag, and took thence a stone, and slang it, and smote the Philistine in his forehead, that the stone sunk into his forehead; and he fell upon his face to the earth.

I noticed Lonnie's breathing had leveled out. Mary came in and she saw it too. She told me Lonnie was breathing easier.

That was on Friday, May ninth. Lonnie Simmons died on the following Tuesday. I didn't get the news until Thursday. I called Lonnie's number, hoping I would be able to talk to Mary. I didn't know Mary's phone number on Cox Street, and she wasn't listed in the telephone book. Nobody answered the telephone at Lonnie's, so I left a message expressing my sympathy. It didn't occur to me to look up Jo-Anne Simmons's telephone number. I could have called Jo-Anne. As it turned out, Hospice didn't notify me when the funeral would be held, nor did I look through the obituaries in *The Opelika-Auburn News*. I later learned that the funeral had taken place on Saturday, May 17th, at Shiloh A.M.E. Zion Church, in Opelika.

I did send Mary a condolence card, at Lonnie's address. I intended to call Jo-Anne Simmons; through Jo-Anne I could arrange to meet with Mary. But the thought of picking up the telephone brought back the tiger-striped rims of Jo Anne's sun glasses. I ended up not calling her.

Over two months later, early in August, the new director of Hospice volunteers, Linda Merritt, gave me Mary Wagner's telephone number. When she heard my voice, Mary responded with pleasure. She said she would like to see me. She had a doctor's appointment tomorrow, and on Friday she had to do housework for this lady, and Saturday was her church meeting day. Then she asked me for my telephone number. I pushed a little—you tell me when it's convenient, I said to her, and I'll come over and see you. She said she would call me next week.

A week went by. Mary Wagner didn't call me. I didn't hear from her until Christmas. She wrote a note on a Christmas card (I had also sent her a Christmas card), saying how much she had appreciated talking to me. In the note, she said there were times when she still felt low. She asked me to call her, she'd like to take me out to lunch sometime.

I telephoned her a few days later and right away she said she'd like to take me out to lunch. I put her off, yes, let's do it next week, something like that. During our conversation, she didn't bring up having lunch again. She did say she was getting along pretty well. She thanked me again, and I said I was glad I could be with her. Then I was sitting with the receiver in my hand.

I tried to recover my image of her. A middle-aged African-American woman, a little overweight, that was what came back to me. Then I remembered Mary sitting out with Jo-Anne on the front porch, the sunlight gilding leaves in the pecan tree, smoke ribboning up from Mary's cigarette.

3

"He Served under General Patton . . . and General Eisenhower"

I STARTED SEEING Howard Carr on June 13, 1998, about a month after Lonnie Simmons died. In the interim some changes at Hospice had come about. Hospice had moved to a big new building on Opelika road, sharing office space with Lee County Home Care. A new position was created for Bill Wanamaker, Director of Public Relations. Linda Merritt became the new Director of Hospice Volunteers. I'd already met Linda Merritt at a breakfast for Hospice volunteers, but we hadn't had a chance to talk much. She did tell me she'd taught freshman comp at the Opelika branch of Southern Union Junior College. Grading endless sets of themes, I rejoined, I'd done that myself once.

On Friday morning she called me to tell me she had a new patient for me. He had a brain tumor, but he wasn't that bad off yet. We arranged to meet in her office, on Monday morning at ten. I parked in a space marked Visitors, in a large horseshoe-shaped parking lot. I walked up a concrete ramp instead of taking the steps, and, entering, told the woman at the front desk I was here to see Linda Merritt. She directed me to the first office to my right. Leaving the reception room, I passed photographs of deceased patients, a copying machine, and a loaded-up cork bulletin board. I took the first right to Linda's office.

A petite woman in her thirties was waiting for me behind a cluttered desk. She was wearing a pale gray summer suit, her white blouse open at the neck. Her pale blond hair, pulled tightly back, was held in place with a butterfly shaped barrette. Linda got up and held her hand out, creating enough space between us so we could interact in a casual way without getting chummy. Shaking hands with her, I said it was good to see her again.

We didn't stay long in her office. Linda stopped off in the reception room up to pick up a Hospice documentation sheet and a set of car keys. There was something resolute in the way she carried herself. She led me to a white Pontiac, unlocked the door from the driver's side, got in, then reached over to flip the lock on the passenger's side. I got in, and Linda started the car. She turned the air on, and while the car was cooling off, she entered the mileage on the documentation sheet, along with the time of departure.

The Carrs lived south of Opelika, off U.S. 169. That was a good ten miles from Auburn. It took us about half an hour to get there. On the way, Linda told me she had an M.A. in English at Mississippi State, with a creative thesis in poetry. She had done her undergraduate work at Mississippi State College for Women, where she had majored in English and started writing poetry.

I asked her if she was still writing. She told me that she hadn't written any poetry for some time. She went on to say how important validation was for a writer, for how else can you know whether you're any good or not. She told me she'd met Nikki Giovanni at a writers' conference in Mississippi. Nikki Giovanni had asked Linda to send her some poems, and had written her back how much she liked them. That was validation, I said. "Yes, but I didn't write her back," she said, "I was too much in awe of her, I suppose."

We had no trouble finding the place. The Carrs lived in a doublewide, one of several along the last stretch of road. Their place was just beyond an orange pylon, and behind that, the blacktop road reached a dead end. Imprinted on the aluminum mailbox was the name CARR, and in the center of the sun-drenched front yard stood a stone angel bordered with rocks, hands clasped in prayer, in a tiny grove of spiky palmettoes. Not far from the stone angel were two metal lawn chairs upholstered in floral magenta, with a low, round table in front. There seemed little likelihood of their being put to use. There was a school bus along the left border of the big front yard, seventy or eighty feet away from the house. It had curtains in the open windows, and the paint was chipped and faded.

The windows of the doublewide had dark blue shutters, and the front steps were carpeted in a prickly, incandescent green Astroturf.

Helen Carr met us at the door. A woman in her sixties, she was close to my height, much taller than Linda. Her hair had turned gray and she was getting stout; yet her face had retained a youthful sweetness. When Linda introduced me, Helen Carr's eyes showed mistrust until, smiling, pitching my voice in a downhome mode, I said, "nice to meet you, Mrs. Carr."

Helen smiled and we shook hands, and then she led us through the front parlor into the living room—chalk blue wall to wall, console TV, a sofa, a big armchair, paneled walls. We sat down, made ourselves comfortable. She told us her husband was asleep; he had been sleeping a lot lately. I said to Helen I'd heard her husband was in the military—Linda had already informed me of this. That was something Helen could talk about. She pointed out a large map of France and western Germany, on one wall above a fireplace, with red dots marking battle sectors from Normandy on beyond the Rhine. I had a glimpse of a framed photograph, an enlisted man wearing summer khakis and a garrison cap with a broad bill. Helen went on to say her husband had been in the 102nd Cavalry Command. I asked Helen what general he'd served under, and she said, "He served under General Patton." She paused, reflecting on what she'd said, and added "and General Eisenhower, he was Supreme Commander."

We stayed in the living room a little longer. Helen told us they had just come back from a trip. They'd gone back to where her husband had grown up, in a small town in southeastern Georgia, about fifty miles south of Savannah. She said her husband's condition had worsened since then. Then, a little stiffly, "we feel we accomplished what we set out to do." A voice resonated out of a speaker on one wall, a nasal babbling, peremptory in tone. I couldn't understand what was being said. Helen said she would be right there. She moved across the room toward the bedroom door, pausing to signal us to follow her.

His head propped up on three pillows, Howard Carr was stretched out on one side of a king-size bed. He was wearing a T-shirt, and light blue jeans that left his veined ankles exposed. His feet were bare, toes pointed inward. He had a hooked nose, a bald head, big thick-lobed ears, thin lips. On the dresser, to the right of the bed, was a color photograph of Howard and Helen, Howard filling out his dark blue double-breasted suit, a big man married to a big woman. They were holding hands, and both were smiling. Another photograph, this one in black and white, displayed another big man, with a graying mustache, children ranging from eighteen to twelve. "That's Howard's son, Eddie," Helen informed us after Linda Merritt commented on it. The children were Howard's grandchildren. Eddie ran a trucking business in Jackson, Mississippi. The family had gone to Europe last month. They had just gotten back last week.

Howard stared out at us through his hooded eyes, his hands

clasped on his chest. Helen moved to his side and took one of his hands. "Mr. Rose is here to keep you company. He's from Hospice. And this is Linda Merritt. She's been very helpful to us."

After Helen finished making the introductions, Howard held out his hand, taking mine with a slow formality the way the very old still do in the South. He let his hand lie in mine a moment.

"Pleasedtomeetcha," he said, running the words together.

He lowered his hand to the bed, without moving his legs or his other hand, his head still propped on the pillow. He must have been waiting for what I might do next, for he kept his right eye shut for awhile. I tried to think of something to say that would interest him.

"I understand you were in the Second World War."

"YesIwas," Howard slurred back at me. "Didmywifetellyou that?"

"She told me you served under General Patton."

"Yesgeneralpatton." And, repeating what Helen had said, only in one slurred rush. "Andgeneraleisenhower."

Now both of Howard's eyes were fixed on me. "Were you in the service?" he asked, not running the words together this time.

I said I had served in the Army three years, not long after the Korean War. He didn't say anything to that.

Linda Merritt moved closer to Howard. She asked him if he enjoyed his trip, going back to his home town in Georgia. He said he did, and looked over at Helen. Helen picked up on that right away, and I could tell Howard Carr liked what he heard. Helen talked about taking their grandchildren to the school Howard had gone to as a boy. She told this funny story about him showing his grandchildren the school house window which, in a moment of childhood rebelliousness, he had thrown an eraser out of. When the teacher came down on him for doing that, Howard had climbed out of the window and run home to his mother. Helen looked over at Howard and smiled. He had enjoyed telling his grandchildren that story.

"Yesthatsright," Howard Carr said.

"You remembered every bit of what happened in the school-house," Helen teased. "But you didn't remember what your mother did when you got home. You may not want to remember that part."

Apparently, Howard didn't, for he closed one eye, then the other. We didn't stay much longer. Before we left the bedroom I got Helen's telephone number. It was on her younger son Roger's business card:

Automotive Equipment and Service.
490 Lee Road 355 Opelika, Alabama 36801
"Specializing in Hydraulic Lifts,
Paint booth … Air Compressors."
ROGER CARR (334) 745-3321

I wrote my telephone number on another one of Roger's cards, and we arranged for me to come back in three days, on Thursday morning from ten to twelve. Helen said mornings were better, for her husband had lunch around noon. He took a nap afterwards.

I turned to Howard. "I'll see you Thursday," I said to him. Howard looked up at me. "Okedoke," he said to me, nodding his head.

Once we were standing at the front door, I asked Helen about the school bus in the yard. It was something to talk about on the way out. Helen had bought it from the City of Opelika, along with several sewing machines for this little business of hers. She told us she was using it to store the fabric she used and the sewing machines. Marking time on the Astroturf, I listened to Helen tell us she sewed up vandalized school bus seats, what the kids did to them on their way home from school. Linda Merritt listened patiently while I looked off at the school bus itself. The area around it was trashed up, lengths of shiny aluminum cylinders, concrete blocks, paint buckets, a section ladder lying flat on the grass. Through the door I made out stacks of fabric. A breeze stirred a set of curtains in the window closest to the road.

From the Hospice Initial Date Sheet:

> History: Recently diagnosed CT Scan of head, 2 tumors.
>
> Description of Present Status: A white elderly male. In apparent distress, denies any pain, nausea, able to ambulate . . . use of rt. leg, wife supportive, understands terminal diagnosis . . . supportive of hospice philosophy.

Three days later I was back to see Howard Carr. Helen had left a message on the answering machine. We would have to change the time because Howard had a doctor's appointment on Thursday morning. When I called her back, she answered listlessly: "Automotive Equipment Service." After I identified myself, her voice brightened up, and we arranged for me to come over on Thursday at 4 P.M.

Since I was a Hospice volunteer and not a chaplain, I felt called upon to read something to Howard Carr besides the Bible. The night before I had finally settled on reading from *Huckleberry Finn*. In reading aloud to a terminally ill white man, I would be using the N word quite a lot. How would Howard respond to that? Certainly not with an African-American's indignation, more likely with an uneasy recognition that the N word had been anathematized. And it was unlikely that he would be aware of the ironies inherent in Huck's attitude toward Jim or the flaws in Huck's own character. What decided me was Helen's story about a boy climbing out of a schoolhouse window after pitching an eraser out. That experience still meant something to Howard Carr. So *Huckleberry Finn* might bring back a time when he was a rebellious young boy, which should be "an enhancement of life," as we Hospice people would term it, for the two hours I would be reading to him.

On Thursday afternoon on my way to the Carrs', I took Lee 412 out of Auburn. It was a warm day in May, heaps of cumuli, a cobalt sky. For half a mile or so, kudzu-mantled trees, kudzu draped on a telephone line, sedate country homes set back on large front lawns, pastures, a private lake, low rises opening out ahead, sloping descents to a four-way-stop intersection, red light flashing, slow down, stop. I looked over at the drab concrete block structure to the left—Furniture Restored, Stripping, Caning, Refinishing, a "yes we're open" sign on the closed front door—then to the right at a convenience store with new gasoline pumps, identified by a rebus, LA-Z-followed by a grinning, cartoon bumblebee. A few miles farther at the second stop light, at an Exxon station on my left, I came across an ithyphallic red-coned rocket, the letters FIREWORKS limned from root to tip. There was a shed off to one side, another sign booming out FIREWORKS and NO SMOKING. On my right was a watermelon and tomato stand, in an open trailer behind a panel truck. A black woman wearing a dark blue baseball cap glanced at me dubiously as I slowed to a stop. She must have known I wasn't about to buy a watermelon from her.

Once I passed the second stop light, I wasn't that far from U.S. 169. About two miles from U.S. 169, I passed a plant nursery on the left. After that, stretches of loblolly pine, barbed wire gates, no trespassing signs, lanes receding into what seemed impenetrable gloom. Lee County Lake on the right, sliver of a fisherman's boat on the lake, thickening kudzu on each side of the road.

Finally, Lee 412 dead-ended at U.S. 169, at a used car lot I hadn't noticed on my first trip out with Linda Merritt. Behind a chain link fence loomed a reassuring sign—DUPREE MOTORS,

INC., TRUCKS, VANS, WHOLESALE PRICES. Marshaled in tight little rows, new vans, new pickup trucks, a few new cars, nothing else immediately in sight. I wasn't that far away now. Off 169 I found Lee 189 going off to the left. Tall poplar trees were crowded close to the road. Then I took a left onto Lee 355, passed an orange pylon, came to the angel in the front yard, the school bus, the green carpeted front steps. I picked up a smudged cloth book bag, felt the bulge made by *Huckleberry Finn*.

Inside, I asked Helen how Howard was doing. How did his trip to the doctor go? Helen told me Howard had lost ten pounds. The doctor had urged her to get him to eat more. She said she would be going out for some things. "I'll bring Howard a hot dog, and just hope he's able to eat it."

Helen went back to the bedroom first, perhaps to tidy up, see that Howard was presentable. Marking time, I felt out of place here, an intruder, tolerated but not really wanted. I even thought about leaving. Then Helen was back at the bedroom door, motioning for me to come in.

A clothes dryer was rumbling away. It sat next to a washing machine, in an alcove across from the bathroom. Howard's head was propped up on pillows, not much change in the way he looked. I sat down in an armchair next to the bed, two feet or so from where Howard was stretched out. His feet were a pasty white, purple veins roping his ankles. His toes were pointed in, as they had been before. From where I was sitting—the chair was positioned on a slant—I had a view of Howard's legs and feet, but I had to turn my head to see his face.

I pulled *Huckleberry Finn* out of the cloth bag, a paperback facsimile of the 1884 edition. I asked Howard if he'd like to have me read from it. He said that was fine with him, and Helen said she thought he'd enjoy hearing me read. She told Howard she'd bring him back a hot dog; would he eat it if she brought him one?

She was standing over him at the foot of the bed, which seemed to take up half of the front yard side of the bedroom. Looking up at her towering over him, he said, "goaheadbring it to me." I was reminded of James Thurber's *New Yorker* cartoons, the implacable, nagging wife, the resentful, long suffering husband, but there was only a hint of Thurber here, in the way Howard kept his eyes trained on her. His eyelids drooped after she left; he seemed to drift off into his own space. The dryer thrummed, the ceiling fan whisked.

I soon realized Howard wasn't interested in carrying on a conversation. So I said if it was all right with him I'd just get started reading. I asked him if he'd ever read *Huckleberry Finn*. He said he had, longtimeago.

I opened the book to the NOTICE, thinking I'd read that first, which I did, with great confidence in the effect I would produce.

NOTICE
Persons attempting to find a motive in this narrative will be prosecuted; persons attempting to find a moral in it will be banished; persons attempting to find a plot in it will be shot.
BY ORDER OF THE AUTHOR
Per. C.G. CHIEF OF ORDINANCE

What I got back from Howard was protracted silence. Okay, I'll go on to the next thing. Let's get untracked, I said to myself.

I turned the page, expecting to see Chapter I. What greeted me was Chapter V. This couldn't be! Something was badly wrong! I flipped back through the long introduction, but found no missing four chapters. It came back to me then. Two years ago I had picked up the book at the Department of English office, one of many used as supplementary reading for a survey course in American lit, EH 270, 271, 272. Was my copy the one bad apple in the barrel? Or did all the copies start with Chapter V? It came back to me, what must have happened. I'd picked this copy under the impression I would be teaching EH 271 that quarter. *Huckleberry Finn* was supplementary reading for EH 271. Later I realized I was teaching third quarter EH 272, from Frost and Hemingway to Raymond Carver. I kept my copy of *Huckleberry Finn* without opening it. Or if I had, I'd forgotten about the missing chapters. Talk about absent-minded professors!

I was unable to speak with Howard staring at me, and I didn't know what to do next. My first thought was to postpone the reading. I would bring something else to read next time. No, Howard was waiting for me to read *Huckleberry Finn*, now, not another book next time. The only thing was to push on. "Well it looks like the first four chapters are missing. I guess we'll have to start with Chapter Five. Is that okay with you, Howard?"

"Itsokay," Howard said quietly.

First I did a summary of what took place before Chapter V. This boy Huck Finn, he lives at the Widow Douglas's place, in a town on the Mississippi. She tries hard to civilize him, make him learn manners and all. Huck runs away from the Widow Douglas because he's sick of all this civilizing. And he's sick of going to school. I went on to characterize Pap because that's where we'd be starting out today. Then, turning away so I was viewing Howard's feet, I cleared my throat and started in.

"Chapter Five. 'I had shut the door to. Then I turned around and there he was.'"

I read some more, then paused to show Howard a pen and ink drawing of a gaunt, scraggly-bearded Pap tilted back on a stool, hands in pockets, one bare foot crossed over the other. Howard looked at it without responding, so I decided I wouldn't show him the illustrations. Yet as I read on I saw that Howard was listening intently. I got to what Pap said about Huck's schooling. "And looky here—you drop that school, you hear. I'd learn people to bring up a boy to put on airs over his own father and let on to be better'n what he is, you hear? Your mother couldn't read, and she couldn't write nuther, before she died. None of your family couldn't, before they died. I can't and here you are a-swelling yourself up like this." Howard let out a tiny harrump of pleasure. Looking up from the book, I saw a smile on his face.

"Huck's pap, he's down on Huck going to school," I said.

"Thasright," Howard said back to me, but what he wanted was more of the book. So I read on, without much comment.

I read five chapters that day, from V through IX. Huck's escape from Pap's cabin, that was a little too complicated for Howard to follow, but his attention picked up when Huck was on the river, making for Jackson's Island. I read about Huck hearing voices, "how far a body can hear on the water such nights,"—something Howard might know from his own experience, or so it seemed from his murmur of assent. And that first day on Jackson's Island, the ferry boat firing a cannon to bring Huck's corpse to the surface, Huck's sudden glimpse of the people he'd left behind, Pap, Tom Sawyer, Becky Thatcher passing by on the ferry, "they could a run out a plank and walked ashore." Howard seemed to be following most of it.

We went on to Huck finding Jim, and for the first time I read out the N-word. It doesn't show up right away. In fact it is not used that much in the early chapters of the novel (Take a look at Sherwood Anderson's "I Want to Know Why"; the N-word is used over twenty five times to show the narrator's confused innocence). Jim himself uses it first. He's in the middle of one of his chuckle-headed bad luck stories, how he was bilked of fourteen dollars by "'dat one-loigged nigger dat b'long to old Misto Brodish.'" I dropped the word in without comment and moved on. Howard didn't comment either. It was as if both of us were silently conceding that the N-word had to be there. But that didn't make us happy about it.

About an hour after I started reading, Howard's younger son, Roger, dropped by. He looked like his brother Eddie, except his mustache wasn't gray. A big, broad-shouldered man, he had on Wrangler shorts and a red polo shirt. He came up to the foot of the bed and asked Howard what the doctor had told him this morning. Howard said he had lost ten pounds. Roger didn't say anything to that. He said he couldn't stay long today, but he'd be back tomorrow and would see Howard then. We shook hands before Roger left. "Appreciate your coming over," Roger said to me.

A little later Helen's sister Caroline came by. She was wearing a baggy print dress that came down below her knees. She looked considerably older than Helen, well into crow's feet and dewlap territory, but she still had a bouncy exuberance. "I bought you a plate of spaghetti and meatballs. You make sure you eat some, Howard." Howard told her he would.

Not long after I got back to reading, Howard told me he had to use the bathroom. I closed the book up and set it aside. I took his elbow to help him get out of bed, and kept him steady while he took short steps into the alcove. He left me outside the bathroom door, pulling it halfway closed. I turned away, hearing him tinkle and grunt in there.

While he did his business, he asked me how many children I had. I said I had two sons and two daughters. I said my eldest son was born in 1960. All of my children were grown up now. Then Howard was standing in the bathroom door, his knees bent, slightly stooped, hiking his jeans up past his thighs, then on up over his jockey shorts, which he must have pulled up in the bathroom. I said I thought his son Roger looked like his other son, the one in the photograph. "That's Ed," he said, "he's my oldest boy. He's in the trucking business." I noticed Howard was no longer running slurred words together. He didn't say anything more. That was the extent of our conversation. Buttoning up, he shuffled back to the bed.

I went back to reading *Huckleberry Finn* to Howard. Sometime later, Helen was back. She had an appreciative smile for me. I put the book back in my bag, and asked her if she had the hot dog; oh yes, it was in the kitchen. She asked me how the reading had gone, and I replied that it had gone pretty well. I told her Roger had stopped by; he had told Howard he would be back tomorrow. Howard didn't say much, but he was listening. All of a sudden Helen asked me where I was from. I told them I'd grown up in Indiana, in Kokomo, north of Indianapolis. I'd gone to college at Vanderbilt University, in Nashville, Tennessee, and done an M.A. and a Ph.D. at the University of Florida, in Gainesville. I'd spent most of my adult life teaching at Auburn University. I didn't go into the why of all of this, yet something compelled me to say that I'd rather live in the South than in the Midwest. The summers were hot but the winters weren't bad, and Southerners, I had discovered, were generally easy to get along with.

Helen said she'd never lived anywhere else but in the South. "I know people say bad things about us down here, but we like it here." She looked over at Howard and said fondly, "He wouldn't live anywhere else."

"Thasright," Howard said, with authority.

I shook hands with him before I left. I said we'd read more when I came back to see him next week.

"Okedoke. See you next week," he said.

ANOTHER VISIT. ANOTHER READING. My chair was positioned

the same way, so that my normal view over the edge of the book encompassed Howard's legs and bare feet. I felt relaxed, at ease being here, with no concerns beyond the present moment. Helen stayed in the living room. She had clothes in the dryer again, and she came in once to take the clothes out. The reading didn't go well this time. Howard kept his mouth open and his eyes mostly closed. At times I wondered if he were awake, but when I said something about what I was reading, looking over to my right at his face, he would open one eye and say something back, not much, enough to let me know he was still there. I thought I might get a smile out of him by demonstrating two ways of threading a needle, what Mrs. Loftus describes in Chapter XI to convince Huck he does "a girl tolerable poor." In his role as Sarah Williams, Huck tries to fit the eye of the needle into the thread instead of poking the thread at the needle. Male and female needle-thread-ers, I went through the motions of each in turn, but Howard's response was no more than perfunctory. The smile he thought he should make died on his lips. I had a sense of relief when Howard told me he'd like to rest now. He moved his left leg in a leisurely way, crossing it over the right.

Helen was watching television in the living room. She turned the set off and we talked a little while. Her fourteen-year-old grandson from Jackson, Mississippi—that was Eddie, Jr.—was due in tonight; he would be staying with them for several weeks. Eddie, Jr. was a good cook, Helen told me, and she knew he would be a lot of help to her. I noticed two photographs on the wall, two wide-eyed, freckled kids on the near edge of adolescence. They were photographs, Helen informed me, of Roger and Ed-die when they were boys. I thought back on myself at that age. I used to ask myself—what, at age thirteen, was I good for, where was I going from here?

Driving back on Lee 355, about to pass two trailers off to my left occupying the same broad swath of acreage, I had to slow down to take it all in—cane pole and bobber, floppy straw hat, patched overalls, nut brown face, another Huck Finn, fishing out of a brick bordered pool not much larger than a bathtub (I couldn't tell whether there was water in it). Was this Jungian synchronicity or some kind of post-modernist mockery, archetype degraded to shoddy gimcrack? No, this black Huck Finn had a down-to-earth charm, he belonged here with the two trailers, even though, here in East Alabama today, there was no territory for him to light out for.

THE LOOK OF THE DOUBLEWIDE had changed. I realized that it hadn't been painted for awhile. The magenta-flowered chairs by the green carpeted front steps had been moved some distance off, to the right of the front yard, under a cottonwood tree, next to three skeletal lawn chairs. A section ladder was planted against the roof, a little to one side of the bedroom.

Inside, I met the grandson, young Eddie Jr. He was sprawled out in an armchair, parked in front of the television set, a thin boy with dark curly hair. I noticed he was wearing braces. Helen didn't have much to say to me this time, just that Eddie Jr. was a big help to her. And, yes, Howard was feeling better. She didn't go with me to the bedroom.

Entering the bedroom, I kept my eyes off Howard, hurrying to the familiar armchair, plopping down in it. Soon I repositioned the armchair so I would be looking at Howard's face instead of his legs and feet. He was wearing the usual T-shirt and jeans, but instead of lying on his back with his head propped up, he lay facing me, his left hand behind his head, his legs dangling over the side of the bed. Before I got started reading, I asked him how he was feeling.

Right away, he said, "Feelenbetter."

The next thing to ask was easy, for I remembered he was supposed to put on weight. "Have you been eating better lately?"

"YeahandI'mtakingatonic."

Once again I commenced reading. When something funny
took place in the novel, Howard would smile, and something like
a twinkle would come into his eyes. Chapters XV and XVI he
attended to with considerable seriousness. In Chapter XV, Huck
tricks a grieving Jim into thinking he dreamed they were separated
in the fog. Then, seeing leaves and rubbish on the raft, Jim realizes
they *have* been separated. He tells Huck what he thinks of him.

> "En when I wake up en fine you back agin', all safe en soun',
> de tears come en I could a got down on my knees en kiss yo'
> foot I's so thankful. En all you wuz thinkin 'bout wuz how you
> could make a fool uv ole Jim wid a lie. Dat truck dah is trash;
> en trash is what people is dat puts dirt on de head er de fren's
> en makes 'em ashamed."

Jim gets up slow and goes into the wigwam, and Huck says
he could have almost kissed Jim's foot to get him back. "'It was
fifteen minutes before I could work myself up to go and humble
myself to a nigger—but I done it, and I warn't ever sorry for it
afterwards, neither.'"

Howard's eyes showed the message had gotten through to
him. I felt we had come away with something we might not
have thought of for awhile. The very familiarity of these reread
words, our recognition of them yet one more time may have come
through to both of us.

But it wasn't long before Howard lost interest. I caught him
dozing, or looking as if he were, while I read on. No, not quite,
he perked up as the raft passed Cairo and Jim lost his chance to
gain his freedom. I think Howard sensed what that meant for a

fugitive slave. But by the time we got to the Grangerfords, and in particular as I read Huck's description of the Grangerford house, I realized Howard had been read to enough for one day. We'd pick up next time where we left off. I left him lying in bed, propped up with pillows, his hands folded, about to drift off to sleep.

OUTSIDE THE TRAILER, on the near side of the carpeted steps, Helen was weeding a zinnia and marigold bed with a garden trowel. A yellow garden hose stretched from a spigot next to the section ladder. She saw me approaching and called out to me. "Go on back, Mr. Rose." The last time I was here she had called me Mr. Ross. I hadn't said anything to correct her. This time she had the name right.

Eddie Jr. was sitting in front of the television set. He might have been rooted there since the last time I was here. I said hello and he nodded at me. I went on back to the bedroom.

Howard was wearing clean white jockey shorts, hanging loose on his loins. A skimpy brown-checked sheet covered his chest, looped his buttocks, wound around one leg. For the first time I noticed the plum-colored liver spot along his right wrist. With his right hand he was trying to rearrange the sheet so it would cover his legs from his knees to his groin. Then he gave up on the sheet, and lay back clasping his hands. By that time I had positioned the chair, angling it so that, looking up from my book, I wouldn't be seeing the sheet, the jockey shorts; no, I would stay focused on Howard's clipped toenails. The chair I sat in was a ladderback chair, not the armchair, which had been moved next to the dryer. Now it was heaped with folded clothes and towels.

Leaning forward as Helen came in, I realized my polo shirt was stuck to the back of the chair. I made a lunge and it crackled loose.

From the foot of the bed, Helen said, "While Mr. Rose is reading I'm going to take the garbage out and go get some gasoline for the mower."

Howard mumbled something undetectable. Then Helen was out the door. I wondered who was going to mow the yard. Most likely, Eddie Jr. That would get him away from the television set.

Not much got read that afternoon. Howard lay with the sheet draped over his chest and belly, his thin arms cradling his lolling head, his eyes blank, while I droned through the Grangerford/ Shepherdson feud. I was just getting used to seeing him that way when, abruptly, he swung his feet around, got himself sitting on the edge of the bed, rearranging the sheet in the process. I stopped reading, leaning forward in the pesky ladderback, stripping off my adhesive-edged shirt again. The blank look went out of his face and he quit fussing with the sheet.

Howard was first to speak. He said it was hot today. I agreed, but since the ceiling fan and floor fan were cooling the room, I felt I could say it wasn't that hot in here. We talked a little longer about the heat. After pausing to think of what to say next, I asked him how long he and Helen had lived here.

"Eightyears," he quickly came back.

Another pause, silence flooding in. Then I asked him where he lived before they moved here.

"Andalusia. It'sreallyhotthere."

I couldn't think of anything more to say to him, yet we couldn't just silently look at each other. So I offered to draw him a picture. Would he like that?

"Thasfine."

I tore off a page from a notebook I carried with me, and got out a black felt-tip pen. I drew a jut-jawed right handed hitter, a squatting catcher behind home plate, and with respect to authenticity I remarked, "Let's see, the catcher's mitt is in the left hand." Howard had no reply to make. I put some spectators in the background, added a fast ball nearing home plate. Leaning forward, I turned the drawing so Howard could have a look at it.

"It's a ball game. There's a guy at bat. You can't see the pitcher but there's the ball. I know it's not a great picture, but anyway it's a picture."

Howard came back, "It'sbetter'nnothin'atall."

"Yes, you're right about that."

Later that afternoon, we talked about the lawn. I was standing up while he was sitting down because he wanted to know if Helen was back. I looked out the window. Helen's Ford Escort station wagon wasn't out there.

"I don't think she's back yet."

I went on to say, "You have a big front yard out there."

"Prettygoodsized."

That ended our conversation.

I was listlessly reading *Huckleberry Finn* to Howard when Helen came back. I watched her go out to the mailbox and come back, leafing through the mail. I wondered how much of it was junk mail.

By this time the feud had run its course. The Grangerford family had been decimated. Huck had witnessed Buck Grangerford and his cousin Joe being riddled with Shepherdson bullets. I was launching into the next chapter—Huck and Jim reunited and back safe on the raft again—when Howard swung out his legs, sitting up again. He looked at his wristwatch, face up on the underside of his wrist. I checked my own watch. I'd spent an hour here and saw no way I could be here much longer today,

"Do you want me to stop reading?"

"Thasfine."

"We'll pick up where we left off next time."

About that time Helen came in. She sat down on the side of

the bed. She took Howard's hand, disregarding the sheet draped like a bath towel over Howard's knees.

I said I'd be out of town early next week, but I'd call her when I got back. Helen said that would work out well for her. She'd had her sister's family to feed last week, and she expected Eddie's family early next week. They were driving over from Jackson, and, on their return trip, they would take Eddie Jr. back with them. That left her two days between visits. "All the food to cook and the dishes to wash." She said Eddie Jr. helped her with the cooking, but she still had to lay in groceries.

I asked her where she did her grocery shopping. Food World, in east Opelika, she said. She took U.S. 169 to the fork just before you got to Uniroyal, that was the short cut to the shopping plaza off U.S. 280. "And there's M . . . M grocery not far down the road. Sometimes I pick up a few things there because he tells me to." She looked fondly at Howard, "I shouldn't be driving that much. He tells me I can't see good."

She patted his hand, but he didn't immediately confirm what she'd said.

Then, "Thasrightyoucan't," he confirmed it.

I realized Helen wasn't in any hurry for me to leave. I asked her who was going to mow the yard, and she said Eddie Jr. would see that that got done, or Roger might come do it this weekend. We talked about living in the country. I said something about subdivisions, that even expensive houses might all look alike with maybe ten feet between them.

"We don't have that here," said Helen, beaming back at me. She told me they never had to lock their doors. The neighbors out here all knew one another. I asked her about the chain link fence across the road. To keep the dogs out of their vegetable garden, she said. We were well into cozy commonplaces, and Howard seemed to be quietly taking it in. His hands were locked below his knees, and he kept a smile on his face. It was as if whatever we said was all right with him.

All at once he was on his feet. And the sheet was no longer with him.

"IsayI'mleavin'!" Just like that.

He did these mincing twinkletoe steps, his body swaying, keeping his balance somehow. He was out the bedroom door in a few seconds. Now Helen and I were on our feet. "He's restless. He's getting up all the time."

I followed Helen out of the bedroom. We found Howard sitting on the sofa, next to Eddie Jr. Side by side, shoulders touching, a smile on his face, an emaciated, nearly finished man was taking delight in his grandson. Eddie Jr. was no longer in front of the TV set. His attention was all for his grandfather now.

I took Howard's flimsy right hand in mine. "See you next time," I said.

"Nexttime."

I don't know why I shook hands with the boy. As I did so, his face lit up. Perhaps he sensed that I was aware of how much his grandfather needed him right now.

I WAS GETTING OUT of my car again, in the heat of a July afternoon. The grass still hadn't been mowed, but the section ladder was back in its place, behind the school bus, almost out of sight. I had a pocket anthology of Robert Frost's poems, thinking Howard might like a change. I'd read "Mending Wall," or "Birches," or "The Road Not Taken."

Coming in through what I now realized was a front parlor, I saw that Helen had Howard in a wheelchair. Last night when I'd called to move my visit up from one PM to two, Helen had told me Howard had had a seizure the night before. Now, she said, he was restless most of the time. But, thank God, she added, he was not in pain.

Helen kept the wheelchair in motion, almost imperceptibly idling it back and forth.

Howard was wearing jockey shorts and a T-shirt. He had a bandage, frayed and spotted with blood, on his right arm above the elbow. He must have been getting some shots. His fingers twitched on the arm of the chair. It came over me, looking into his face, how bad off he was.

I did read "Mending Wall," but Howard wasn't able to follow it. Good fences make good neighbors. Yes, Helen acknowledged, that might be true, but she couldn't keep up the pretense that things were how they were last time. I realized Helen must have been pushing that chair for hours. I offered to take over, "Here why don't you let me do that," I said. She let me take over right away. She told me she had been moving Howard from his bedroom out through the living room and back again. He had kept her up most of the night and part of the morning. "You can't keep on doing this," I said to her. She looked at me and in a level voice said, "I'll just have to take it as it comes." Then she let me take charge of the wheelchair.

I started moving Howard along, at a slow pace, into the kitchen-dining room. The refrigerator door clicked shut as Helen moved to the gas stove with a package of hamburger meat. Helen had help coming this evening, her brother and sister-in-law. "Believe me, he can handle Howard." Her voice had taken on a liveliness now. "My brother will take over the bedroom. And his wife will take over the kitchen. So I know I can get some rest. Howard's brother, if and when he ever comes, he's not going to be much help. He and his wife, they expect to be served."

"They expect to be treated like family," I said.

"Yes, and then some," she said, with a smile.

Leaving Helen in the kitchen, I wheeled Howard back to his bedroom. I could look down at Howard's bald head, note the crosshatched welts on the back of his neck. He seemed almost weightless in the wheelchair.

Turning into the bedroom was a little difficult, for it was necessary to take a diagonal left. First his right foot had to clear the right side of the door, then his left elbow had to clear the door's left side. Howard drew his elbow in, as if away from a fire; he didn't want to get it jammed up in the door. I made sure we had clearance on both sides. I took my time maneuvering the wheel chair in.

We did the bedroom, then went back to the living room, then the front parlor, then the kitchen-dining room. We did the tour nine times. Pushing Howard along, I realized how the house was laid out. I hadn't been in the kitchen-dining room before. It was a sun soaked, pleasant warmish place, with appliances, microwave, dish washer. On the other side, the dining room table was set for six. We passed Helen frying up hamburger meat. On our fourth or fifth circuit we were interrupted temporarily. As we came out into the living room, I recognized Melissa and Virginia, the two black women I'd met while I was with my first Hospice patient, Lonnie Simmons. They'd come to change Howard's sheets and bathe him.

They recognized me right away—you were at Lonnie's; yes, I said, I was. I'd gone out to the porch while they'd done their work. I told them I was sorry I'd missed Lonnie's funeral, I hadn't been notified in time. Seeing me there with Howard, they withheld whatever judgment they might have had. "There are clean sheets in the bedroom," Helen said to Melissa. Howard and I resumed our tour.

We did three or four more circuits while Melissa and Virginia made the bed. Then I turned Howard over to them—they would ease him back onto his bed—and went to join Helen in the kitchen-dining room.

She had the hamburger meat in a skillet. She was having lasagna for dinner, that would do just fine for her guests. I offered to go to the living room so she could have some time to herself, and she said she could cook while we talked. She was standing off from me, in front of the gas stove, prodding hamburger meat with a spatula while I idled in a kitchen chair. The window unit didn't carry this far, but the nodding fans kept it fairly cool. Sunlight came in from several windows, a nice change from the living room's gloom.

Soon Melissa and Virginia popped in; they had the sheets changed and Howard in bed. They'd be back in three days to do it all again.

Helen asked me if I knew anything about brain tumors. I said I didn't. Maybe the nurse could tell you something, or someone at Hospice, possibly, I offered. No, they don't tell you anything about what to expect. One thing—Helen had to tell me this—he's exposing himself, that's a part of it. He'd never do that if he wasn't ill. I asked her when her brother was coming in. Not till this evening, she told me. I said I could come back later this afternoon or stay on awhile if necessary. No need, her son Roger would be back at five. He lived next door—I hadn't realized that. The frame house next door was Roger's.

About that time there was a knock on the door. Before Helen could answer it, she had guests. Her minister, Randall Darby, and his wife Della had stopped by. They looked about the same age, in their early thirties, I guessed, and each of them had put on some weight. They wore clean shorts and open-collared, short-sleeved shirts.

I sat with Della Darby in the living room while Randall Darby and Helen sat with Howard. Right away Della asked me what church I attended. I told her I went to the Episcopal church. She asked me where it was located. I said there were two in Auburn, one downtown, one in the south part of town. I said I'd been to both of them, not saying I hardly ever went to either church anymore.

It wasn't long before Randall Darby and Helen came out. I went back to be with Howard. They stayed in the living room, chatting, what in deep South parlance is called visiting. I got a look at Randall Darby through the bedroom door, on the sofa, knees up, spare tire visible, and beside him his better half, Della. Then I turned to do something for Howard, sit with him, be there for him. It was useless to try to read to him. Howard tried to sit up on the side of the bed. He couldn't even get his shoulders up. He'd raise his head a few inches and give up.

His voice came, needful, bewildered, and I listened and tried to say something back.

"Doggone it!," he said.

"Lordy," I said.

"Doggone."

"I know, Howard. I know it's hard on you."

Then I was sitting beside him, on the edge of the bed. I tried to slip a pillow behind his neck without cracking the lolling, eggshell head. I felt his damp T-shirt next to the palm of my hand. He tried to pick at the blood spotted bandage.

"Doggone."

"I know. It's a damned shame."

Just trying to raise his head, no chance to do that anymore. "Lordy. Lordy have mercy."

"I know I know," I said. "It's a doggone shame."

I took his left hand, felt it warm within mine, but within seconds he was working it loose again. I got up and tried to move his legs. "You need to sleep. Here let me move your legs." They felt heavy, hard for me to lift, but I got them back where they were supposed to be. He was quiet when the social worker came in, a nice-looking, well-dressed young black woman. She took charge, and I was able to go.

I CAME BACK THREE DAYS LATER. I'd given Helen a call before I came. She'd moved the time forward, to 3:30, so my time wouldn't overlap with the women who were coming to bathe Howard. She went on to tell me, "he's declined since you saw him last." He was very weak now, and didn't say much. "But he can hear you, he knows you are there."

Arriving, I saw a young woman next door, driving a lawn tractor. She wore a sleeveless plaid shirt and tight shorts—Roger's wife surely. She was mowing her own back yard. I soon realized that she was mowing the Carr yard also, for there was a swath of mown grass alongside the school bus to my right. Helen's blue Ford Escort station wagon was parked outside in the blistering heat.

Helen told me that the bathing women had come late, so again we sat in the living room, talking sporadically while Melissa and Virginia did their work in the bedroom. Howard's blood pressure was way up and his heartbeat was over one hundred. He did talk some and he knew you, and no he wasn't in any pain. It would be all right if you read to him, Mr. Rose. I said I'd read from the Bible this time.

"I'll stay with him if you want to go anywhere."

"No, I'll stay. I want to be near him," she said.

Helen asked Melissa straight out—how long will he last? Melissa asked her if he'd had his medicine today. Helen hadn't been able to give it to him. Melissa pondered that a moment and then said there was no way she could predict on that today. "We'll have to see how he is Wednesday."

Virginia said he was giving out fast. "But it's hard to tell when someone's ready to go."

They were still there talking to Helen when I went on back to the bedroom.

Howard didn't have the blood stained bandage on his arm, and he wasn't wearing the jockey shorts, but some kind of cloth, perhaps a shirt or a towel, partially covered him. With the fingers of his left hand he was fumbling in his exposed crotch. His mouth was open; so were his puckered eyes. Sometimes he raised his left arm, then back it went to where it wanted to be, and the fingers were plucking and pulling. His breath rasped out while he moved his hand. Helen came in only once. She slipped the cloth out from under his buttocks, folded it, and set it between his legs. I went on reading how David slew the Philistine Goliath while she did that, and then, without a word to me, she left me with him.

I read from the Gospel According to St. Matthew, on through half of the Sermon of the Mount, pausing between verses. And then from the Psalms, I read a few Psalms at random and then the Twenty-Third Psalm. Then I read the first two books of Genesis. I think Howard was able to follow some of it. Throughout most of my reading, Roger's wife, behind the wheel of a riding lawn mower, was mowing the front yard. She had already mowed the front yard next door. Periodically, the deafening roar of the mower interrupted my reading. Once, the din receding as I read the serpent's seduction of Eve, Roger's wife lifted her hand to her hair. Not long after Adam partook of the forbidden fruit, I heard thunder rolling in from the east. The room darkened, and a wind started up. I saw the tops of the trees across the road shuffling, and heard the window frames creak, the windows rattle.

Finally, I had to stop reading. Howard Carr remained mute. I laid one hand on Howard's wasted arm and said it was time for me to go.

I telephoned Helen on Friday, to work out a time for my visit and tell her I couldn't come over next week, for I was flying to Indiana to spend a few days with my brother. We had planned this get-together two months ago; I had already paid for my ticket. I told Helen I would ask Linda Merritt to send another volunteer if that's what she wanted. Helen said she would think about it. She'd have family with her, and now that Howard was in such a bad way, there wasn't much a volunteer could do. But she did want to see me this afternoon. I said I'd get there around two, but something came up, and I was half an hour late.

It rained hard on my way out. By the time I got there the rain had stopped. I picked my way past soggy patches in the front yard. I noticed Helen's station wagon wasn't parked out front. Roger's wife Barbara greeted me. She had her daughter Staci with her, a shy ten-year-old.

The three of us went back to the bedroom. Staci stayed near the door, her eyes on the man stretched out on the bed. Howard was wearing plastic diapers. A tube ran from beneath his buttocks, curling somewhere under the bed. His head was propped on two pillows, his left leg dangling over the edge of the bed. The brown-checked sheet I'd seen before was snarled up around his ankles and calves.

Barbara hoisted his left leg, set it back on the bed. "Mr. Rose is here to read you something," she said.

Howard said something, I couldn't make it out, his voice parrot-like, disconcerting. Barbara reached over and untangled the sheet, spreading it deftly over his legs. "I'll leave you with him," she said to me, before she and Staci left the bedroom.

I sat down on the ladder back, and opened the Bible to Genesis. "And it came to pass, when they were in the field, that Cain rose up against Abel his brother, and slew him." Howard seemed to take no notice of me. He moved his left hand to different places, his chin, his navel, the crinkled plastic, pushing at it with the tips of his fingers. Or his hands were folded on his chest. He was breathing easily most of the time.

I would read a little, then pause to gaze out the window, at the angel in the front yard, rain-washed, fringed with palmetto leaves, the Venetian blind slats segmenting my view. I'd watch the fan going, notice it rattling a little, scrutinize folded clothes, the brown checks in the sheet, Howard's trimmed toenails.

We played out this comedy, the left-leg comedy. I think Howard knew damned well what he was doing, although at first I didn't think so. His left leg sliding off the edge of the bed, I'd seen Barbara pick it up and put it back where it belonged. So I did the same thing she did. I'm not sure why. Perhaps I really wanted do something for him; or did I just want to be doing something physical. I tried to tell myself—forget about Howard's leg.

I got to Noah, the ark, the flood. Something minute in the text got my attention. "Of every clean beast thou shalt take to thee by sevens, the male and his female, and of the beasts that are not clean by two, the male and the female." I read the next verse. "Of fowls also of the air by sevens, the male and the female; to keep seed alive upon the face of all the earth." The unclean beasts, which ones were they? Howard's left leg slid off the bed for the third or fourth time. This time, when I tried to put it back, after setting the Bible, place marked, on the chair, the leg resisted me, it wouldn't budge. I realized Howard didn't want me to move his leg.

"All right, if that's how you want it," I said to him, "I'll leave your leg right where it is." After that he moved his leg up and down himself. It could have been a little dance he was doing. He'd let it slip down and pull it back up. I couldn't go on reading the Bible. I started talking to him with frenetic good cheer, spewing out nonsense, how we had a hard rain, how next week I was making this trip to Indiana, how it wasn't the same up there as it is here. I was on my feet, then sitting down again. I read on, came to the covenant. "And I will establish my covenant with you; neither shall all flesh be cut off any more by the waters of a flood; neither shall there any more be a flood to destroy the earth."

I was moving on to Abraham and Isaac when it happened. Howard Carr was turning his body now so he could look up at me, sitting over him now. His eyes were slits, barely open, so he may not have seen me that well. His hands were folded on his chest.

There came this parrot-like squawking gibberish—unmistakably meant for me.

"What is it you want?" I asked him.

One thing. One word. "Leave!"

"Is that what you want? Are you sure?"

"Leaveleaveleave!"

I said good-bye but he didn't respond. Then I did what he wanted, I left.

I talked to Barbara on the way out. I told Barbara that Howard had told me to leave. That didn't surprise her. She said Howard had been difficult lately. That made it easier for me to go. I did ask her to tell Helen I'd be in touch with her when I got back from my trip. Barbara said Helen would appreciate that. Then she told me Helen and Roger had gone to the funeral home to make arrangements in advance.

"They wanted to do it ahead of time." She touched one template of her glasses. "They're afraid things might jam up on them later."

"That's understandable," I said, agreeing all too readily that it was the right thing for Helen to do. I didn't ask whether Howard had been told of this, probably not was my assumption. "I know Helen's been through a lot."

"Yes, it's been an ordeal for her. I don't know how she's been able to manage so well. I know I couldn't. But Helen's been wonderful."

I felt lousy driving back. I should have read to Howard or quietly sat with him, or left early, done something different. Instead I had moved his leg back up on the bed, talked nonsense, read to him in a halfhearted way. I had taken note of his wasted body, nothing I had done had been right. What had happened was irreversible.

"WOULD YOU GO back with me, Helen? I think Howard was mad at me Friday."

"He was mad at everyone Friday."

The next day I came back with three carnations at seventy-nine cents apiece. I didn't stay long this time. Helen went back to the bedroom with me.

A large white sheet covered Howard, not the brown-checked rag I'd gotten used to. The room had a sick room's pallor; the Venetian blinds were closed, dimness everywhere. Helen went over to Howard, held the carnations out for him. "Mr. Rose brought some flowers for you," she said solicitously. She lowered the flowers toward his face. Nothing registered, so she moved them away.

Driving back, not far beyond Lee County Lake, I saw a crow hunched over a slimy carcass. It didn't lift off, flap away like a buzzard; no, it strutted on bird feet across the road.

TWO DAYS AFTER I got back from Indiana, I sat with Helen in the shadowed side of the living room. Howard was asleep in the bedroom. He was sleeping most of the time now, but at night, usually from twelve to two, he'd be agitated; that never failed to happen, Helen said, so someone had to be in bed with him.

She said she hadn't been getting much sleep.

We chatted for over an hour, as if we knew one another better than we did. From time to time I glanced at the map displayed on one wall, the photograph of Howard in khakis attached to the map, but mostly I looked at Helen. We kept eye contact most of the time. What emerges from what she said that afternoon was the strength of Helen's devotion. And how well she had thought out what had to be done.

"You do what you have to do," she said more than once. She was doing that, and taking pride in it.

She told me how she gave Howard his medication, with the same sense of accomplishment Mary Wagner showed when she described how she medicated Lonnie Simmons. Mary had used an eyedropper, learning that technique along with much else. Helen had her own method. At the end of the day she shook out Howard's pills and mashed them up with a tablespoon. She put Saran wrap over the tablespoon, that way she would be able to medicate him right away, whenever Howard became agitated. She stirred the mashed up pills into a bowl of applesauce, spoon-feeding Howard as if he were a baby again, while the daughter-in-law who lived next door or her sister who was visiting held Howard on the edge of the bed. Helen demonstrated the position, contorting herself in the armchair. You had to get behind Howard, scissor Howard with your legs, letting his back lie back against your breasts, but making sure you kept his head up.

"It's like having a baby in the house. That's what I tell my-self."

Helen got up and went to the kitchen. She came back with jars of Gerber liquid baby food—macaroni and cheese dinner, chicken and dumpling dinner, what Howard liked for dinner when he was well, banana, carrots, spinach on the side; eat your cauliflower, I thought, remembering what that had been like when I was a child. I said, I'll bet you don't give him cauliflower.

"That's right. Howard hates cauliflower."

There was a pause, our eyes drifted off. After a little while, we reconnected.

"So in a sense," I said, "you're still cooking for him."

Helen smiled and said, "That's right; I am. But I don't tell him he's getting baby food. My daughter-in-law came out with that once, and he closed his mouth and wouldn't eat any more." Helen tightened her lips, "Eating baby food, that's something he doesn't want to do. So we put Kleenex around the jars, or put the baby food in a bowl for him."

She'd refused to have a hospital bed in the house, even though Hospice had pushed her to take one. That meant she had to put diapers on Howard and take him to the bathroom. But that was something she had learned how to do. He wouldn't want to be in a hospital bed. She couldn't do that herself, that she realized, but she had family to help her out. And the people at Hospice were also a help, in fact without them she couldn't have managed. And she also appreciated my volunteer work. "It's meant a lot, your coming out here."

Before I left I said I'd have a look at Howard. I went back to the bedroom by myself. Howard lay with his head to one side, the black hole of his mouth cranked open, his eyes glued shut. I stayed close to the door, listening to his heavy breathing, waving my left hand back and forth a few times, before I left him there, asleep in his bed.

Howard Carr died the following Sunday, at the age of seventy-four. On Monday morning, I received a telephone call from Lee Merritt. Howard had had a seizure, she said, and had been in considerable pain near the end. Helen hadn't been there to see him die. She'd gone off to do some shopping, leaving Howard with her brother, the brother who, she'd told me earlier, on that first day Howard was so bad off, would be able to "take over the bedroom," while his wife "took over the kitchen."

On Wednesday night I went to Frederick's Funeral Home to be with the family. For a little while. The map, Howard's photograph in khakis was on an easel next to the casket. As soon as Helen saw me, she came over and touched my arm. I went over with Helen to look at Howard one last time. Howard was wearing his blue suit; his face had a waxen repose. Helen and I didn't say anything. She was beside me for half a minute or so. I don't remember much after that; I know I did offer my condolences to the other members of the family.

The funeral was held on Thursday afternoon, in a Methodist church—United Methodist—on the other side of the Beauregard Community School. It would have been a typical country church, weathered clapboard, narrow nave, squat steeple, but this church was broader than it was deep. It did have a graveyard in back, which, as I approached the mourners assembled out front, made me think of Gray's "Elegy In A Country Churchyard." "Some mute inglorious Milton here may rest/ Some Cromwell guiltless of his country's blood."

Country church graveyard images enabled me to get inside the church. Once inside, the air-conditioning blowing calm into me, I sat down in one of the rear pews. Sunlight from the windows on the west side played on the varnished pews. In front of me, several rows of country people. Not all the men were wearing suits, and the women were wearing dresses that had been around for awhile.

An American flag was draped over Howard's coffin, the red and white stripes falling over the side, the square of stars on the casket. Tiers of flowers were on either side of it. The map with Howard's G.I. photograph was also there. Now I was watching Helen enter the church, her sons, their wives, her grandsons, brothers, sisters, a procession of family members filing in behind her to occupy the first three rows of pews. A young woman at a console piano was playing "The Battle Hymn of the Republic." She segued into "Dixie," blending North and South as the last of the family members—brother-in-law, sister-in-law—and many more found their seats. The minister motioned for us to sit down. That was Randall Darby, whom I'd met at Helen's that day Howard was so bad off.

The service itself didn't take that long. Randall Darby not only did the eulogy, which, he said to us, Howard Carr could do without, for his life was testament enough; he sang a hymn, "Peace in the Valley," with feeling and skill. A youngish fluttery blonde girl sang also, "On the Heights" and "I Came to the Garden Alone" while Randall Darby, seated to one side now, looked off into space. He read the Twenty-third Psalm beautifully, and read from the Gospel of John, "Ye will have an advocate, the Holy Ghost." One thing he said about Howard stood out for me—"It's easy to die for Christ but hard to live for Him." The service closed with Randall Darby leading us in singing "Amazing Grace." We sang the first, third, fourth, and fifth verses.

Approaching Helen as I made my way out of the church, at the door with her sons Eddie and Roger, I tried to think of what to say. In its own way it was a lovely service, so that's what I said to her. Her eyes were red, tear-stained; so were her sons' eyes, and their wives. I gave Helen a hug and shook hands with Roger and Eddie. She said to me quietly, "it was good of you to come."

Out of the air conditioning, in the hot August sun, I made for my car in the lot. Something wanted to pull me back, unite me with people I scarcely knew. I took a last look at the church.

A WEEK HAD GONE BY since the funeral. Only the occasional mimosa blossom, no more than a sprig, the trees being laden with drooping pods, some a shiny green, others baked brown. At the second traffic light on Lee 412, the irrepressible fireworks

rocket with the red nose cone was still there, in blast-off position. Across the way, the open trailer, the pickup truck, tomatoes
and watermelons in their bins, tended by the same phlegmatic
baseball-capped black woman, were anchored there for the rest
of the summer. The gate was shut at Lee County Lake, no boats
visible this time. At Dupree Motors, still the shiny new pickups
and vans, but not so many, behind the chain link fence. It didn't
take that long for me to get to the turn, off of U.S 169, a minute,
maybe two went by.

On Lee 355, to my right going in—something was missing
here, something wrong. The trailers were still on the property,
but the black Huck Finn had been carted away, nor was there
water for him to fish in.

Instead, a rock-bordered patch of greenery; how could this be,
white people were living there. A buxom white woman in a tight
pants suit was coming out one of the trailers. So maybe I hadn't
been seeing a black Huck Finn.

Getting out of the car, I heard wind chimes, to the right of me,
where the lawn chairs were grouped in front of the cottonwood
tree. The pallid angel was where I had left it, palmetto bolstered,
in the center of the front yard. The green carpeting on the front
steps threw off glittering particles of light.

Helen and I talked for an hour and a half, in her living room,
without many pauses. At first, she seemed sunk in despondency.
"I'll have to take each day as it comes," she said. But talking made
her feel better.

The bedroom door was shut. Helen's sister, who was still with
her here, was taking a nap in Howard's bed. It would be a viola-
tion of Helen's privacy to elaborate on what we said. I did learn a
few things talking to her. The burial service was held in Howard's
home town in Georgia. He was buried with full military honors.
Two noncoms had come down from Fort Benning to fire the

volleys and present the folded flag to the widow. Taps had been played on a phonograph record.

Helen didn't care for that, unaware that was standard procedure now at most military funerals. Her husband had fought for his country; he had five battle stars; she was convinced he deserved better. I didn't tell her the military had its own rules. Another thing she filled me in on, the American flag was issued at the post office upon receipt of Howard's discharge and separation papers. Her son Eddie had cautioned her to be sure she told the post office people to have the flag pressed. He'd seen some ratty look-ing flags draping coffins. Helen told me it was Eddie's nineteen-year-old daughter who had thought of displaying Howard's map and his photograph in khakis at the visitation and at the funeral. She would never have thought of that herself. Another thing she mentioned, what it cost for an obituary, forty-five dollars. And the paper had gotten the preacher's name backward, Darby Randall, not Randall Darby.

She told me her family would be there for her. She planned to spend November with her sister in Sarasota, Florida, and before that, in September, she'd go to the extended family's annual fish fry in Georgia. She'd spend Christmas with her immediate family in the mountains of northeast Georgia; that Eddie had absolutely insisted on. "He didn't say before Christmas or after Christmas, he said Christmas," Helen said, with a knowing smile.

One thing she knew was this—how pleased Howard would have been at how close the family was. And the funny things that went on, the shared laughter, that too would have pleased him. Her eyes were twinkling as she lost herself in this one story, how they all had a laugh at Eddie, and Eddie too, at himself. Howard would have joined right in, she said. Her son Eddie had carried his beeper around for nearly five days. It was right there in his hip pocket, all during the burial service, and while the preacher was saying the Lord's prayer, in the middle of it, Eddie's beeper went off. Right there in his hip pocket.

"That really threw him," Helen said beaming. I felt my own smile beaming out in accord.

"I'll bet it did. I mean his beeper went off."

"You know what Eddie said later on? He said he was so shook up 'I thought it was divine intervention.' We all had a laugh over that. I know Howard would have too."

Would have? Divine intervention? It seemed like a good time to leave. I knew I wouldn't be back again. I think Helen knew that too. She was still sitting on the sofa as I stood up and held out my hand. She took it and pressed it in hers. "I appreciate all you've done," she said. I tried to thank her for that, but what I did was press my other hand against hers. Then I was walking out through the front parlor, out the front door, down the green-carpeted steps, across the front lawn to my waiting car.

4

Conversations with Eileen Foote

EARLY IN SEPTEMBER, I was assigned a new patient, Cassie Binton, a ninety-three-year-old black woman with esophageal cancer. Linda Merritt gave me a briefing before we paid our visit. Linda was wearing lightweight brown slacks with a check in them, a pale yellow T-shirt, gray stockings and tan oxfords, a pair of wide-framed, sharp-cornered glasses screening her cobalt blue eyes. She was, as usual, very professional. As a Hospice volunteer, I wouldn't be doing that much for the patient, for the care giver, Eileen Foote, had made it clear she didn't need any help. But since Eileen was alone with her aunt almost all the time, she might appreciate having someone to talk to. A young woman in graduate school at A.U. had already been assigned as a volunteer, but she had stopped visiting on a regular basis, claiming her Hospice commitment cut into the time she needed to write her thesis. Linda thought she might have backed out for another reason. Eileen Foote might have been just a little hard for this young woman to take.

"Eileen has some strong opinions," Lee warned me. "And if you give her a chance she'll talk your arm off."

"I'll try not to give her a chance," I said, perhaps too hastily.

Linda's voice softened; she seemed less professional now. "You

might *want* to get to know her. Eileen's not at all disagreeable. All
our people say they like her a lot. The nurses who have tended
Cassie —Cassie's really been shuffled around, I'm afraid—they've
all had good things to say about Eileen."

"I'm sure I'll have good things to say about her too. Once I
get to know her."

Linda smiled. "We'll get started on that today. You'll have me
along to break the ice."

"Yes, that will help."

"I thought it would."

I shifted one leg, waiting for Linda to say something else. She
touched a sharp corner of her glasses. "First thing we have to
do is photocopy an initial data sheet." She pulled the data sheet
out of a folder, got up from her desk, moved to the photocopier.
After scanning the bookcase to my right, taking note of *The Ox-
ford Dictionary of Quotations*, *The Top 500 Poems*, and *Clergy to
Clergy*, I put my mind on what it would be like to be with Eileen
Foote. A black woman, opinionated, garrulous. Mary Wagner,
the last black caregiver I'd been with, hadn't done much talking.
I remembered Mary smoking on her front porch, with Lonnie
Simmons's daughter, Jo-Anne. Neither one of those women would
be smoking a cigarette in Linda's office.

I stood up as Linda came over to my chair. She handed me
the copy she'd made of the Hospice Initial Data Sheet. "Here's
all the info on Cassie's condition," she said crisply. "You can read
it over when you get time."

We left her office and went to the reception area. I read over
the data sheet while she was at the front desk requisitioning a
Hospice vehicle.

Eileen's two children, James and Julia Foote, were also listed
under caregivers. Cassie's church was Community of Jesus of the
Apostolic Faith. Under Description of Present Status I read—"Last

BM8/9. Abd soft. PEG tube site benign. No diff swallowing at present. Lungs clear Pt able to ambulate with assistance. Able to drink water but nutrition is primarily thru PEG."

I asked myself, what does PEG stand for? And the abbreviations, the letters left out, the shorthand necessary to keep the information inside the box meant for it. *Pt had BM 8/9.*

Outside in the parking lot, while Linda went to get the car she'd signed out for, I found I was staring beyond the chain link fence at two arboreal figures in kudzu, draped on face-to-face cottonwood trees, trees leaning into one another as if at any moment they would become animated. A breeze stirred the mass of kudzu, created rustling garments, two women, I thought. I had a print in my bedroom, an etching or lithograph, I don't know which, by Frieda Kohlmeyer—a mother and child leaning into one another, the child's head lowered, her hand out to touch the mother's hand. Through the power of topiary kudzu I felt a sadness out there in the heat of the day. Then Linda pulled the car up, and I got in, leaving topiary mother and daughter behind.

On the way Linda informed me casually that the Foote house wasn't air-conditioned. She had been out this way with Bill Wanamaker to see Eileen Foote several weeks ago. Unintentionally, she led me to believe we might be headed for a place like Lonnie Simmons's house, or a rundown cabin, a shack. Since the heat had let up a little—the highs were down to the mid eighties—I thought I might not need air-conditioning today.

And there was also a dog to contend with. On her first visit with Bill Wanamaker, Linda told me, a redbone hound—Augustine, Eileen had called him—had made a godawful racket outside the car, and Bill had had to honk the horn for awhile before Eileen's son James came around from the back and, calling Augustine off, put him on a leash. Linda pushed her wide-framed glasses up a little, still very much The Director of Volunteers. "James told me Augustine wasn't a mean dog," she said, "but James still put him on a leash."

We took the same road out of Auburn, the road I'd taken so many times to see Howard Carr, Lee 412. We turned right at the second stoplight, leaving the familiar Exxon station behind, the rocket advertising fireworks. This time the rocket was tilted the other way, pointing west not east; one read FIREWORKS backwards and upside down. The tomato and watermelon trailer had vamoosed. After we left Beauregard Community behind (after passing the Methodist church where Howard Carr's funeral service had been held), I took another look at the directions on the Hospice Initial Data Sheet.

"Take Hwy. 51 (towards Hurtsboro) until you see a sign 'Pine Breeze Trailer Ranch,' turn R this is Lee C. Rd 859 follow until dead ends, take L onto Lee Co. Rd. 27, go approx. 2.1 mi, mailbox has # 6221 on it on R house is white black shutters, you may park wherever and enter front door."

Clearly that last sentence had been written by a white person, for under "Living Arrangements and Environment" I read, "Nice older house (well kept)."

It took forty-five minutes for us to get there, for we were actually going out of our way. At Lee 859 we were greeted by a PINE BREEZE TRAILER RANCH sign, with an arrow pointed roughly southwest. At the dead end we turned left on Lee 27. Not many houses on Lee 27, the last leg on our journey—dirt roads pushing through dense pine, some open pasture devoid of livestock, long stretches between the mailboxes. Pine Breeze Trailer Ranch didn't turn up; most likely it was on one of the dirt roads plunging into the pines. At last, on an open patch of land to the right, we reached the mailbox numbered 6221. As we turned in, I looked for the redbone hound, but Augustine wasn't in sight.

"So where is Augustine?"

"Eileen told me Augustine likes to roam around a lot."

"Well that's good. That way you won't have to honk the horn."

"Next time you might have to," Linda said. She collected her purse and we got out of the car.

Eileen met us at the back door, behind a screened-in porch on one side of the house. She was a stout woman wearing a light blue dress that seemed a size or two too small for her. When she smiled, she showed a missing incisor on the left side of her mouth. I got some idea of her character from a quick survey of her kitchen. She had utilized every inch of available space to advantage. The refrigerator top was burdened with cartons of diet cola, boxes of lasagna, spaghetti, various cereals, saltines, cornstarch, cotton balls. To my right, on the kitchen table, were stacked loaves of bread, popcorn, white and brown rice, two bulky Tupperwares containing what looked like a year's supply of flour and sugar. Eileen lived a long way from a supermarket, I thought, and so it made sense for her to load up on staples.

As Linda introduced us, I sensed something uncompromising in Eileen Foote. Yet she was cordial in a formal way. It was evident she wanted us to feel at ease here. We moved on into the living room. Sitting in a rocker by the front window, a young black man in a clean T-shirt and jeans was watching an old AMC black and white '30s movie—elegantly tailored and gowned sophisticates in a penthouse apartment in New York City. A VCR sat atop the television set. Eileen introduced me to her son James, who got up slowly and with a shy formality shook hands with me. Then Eileen took us down a short hall to the back bedroom.

Cassie Binton was lying in a narrow hospital bed with side rails. Her head was turned to the wall. A light blanket covered Cassie's body, from below her feet to just below her neck. Her body made a barely discernible outline, like a shape patted out of sand. She had thick lips, a large flat nose, watery blue eyes. Her cottony hair was plaited. There was a double bed next to the opposite wall. Between the beds, two narrow windows. Drab beige curtains stirred by a fan tilted up from a threadbare rug; closed Venetian blinds tamped down the glare. Standing in the door with Linda, I watched Eileen go to Cassie's bedside. She asked Cassie how she was feeling.

Cassie turned her face toward Eileen, "I have a cold," she said. Her voice was flat, yet it still had strength. Then she was coughing, gagging, clearing her throat.

Eileen turned to Linda Merritt and said, "There's nothing to be done about it. She'll have that coughing until the Lord takes her."

Linda moved toward Cassie and said,. "So nice to see you again, Cassie. You feeling' all right?"

Cassie's slack lips moved. "Not so good today."

Linda introduced me as Mr. Charles Rose, a Hospice volunteer who would be spending some time with her. After Linda made room for me between the two beds, withdrawing to the bedroom door, I went to Cassie and said hello. I said I was glad to meet her and would be seeing her again. Cassie nodded, and let her head slip to one side. Now she was staring at the wall again, at scaly, peeling blue wallpaper, a strip of the stuff hanging from the plaster.

Going out, Eileen said to both of us. "She doesn't have much pain. The Lord blessed her that way, but she's sore."

Eileen left the bedroom door open, and we moved down the hall to the living room. She took a seat in an armchair just off the hall, across from the wall telephone by the kitchen door, and Linda and I sat down on a sofa facing the window. We were sitting across from James, behind a coffee table with a greenish glass top. No sign of a book or a magazine on the coffee table or anywhere else. There were family photographs scattered all over the living room—mostly children, teens, young men and women, all smiling, looking their best. On separate walls, amid the photographs, crocheted letters spelled out PROMISE LITTLE, DO MUCH and GOOD DEEDS LIVE LONG. An open cabinet mounted on one wall was stocked with glass figurines, a gargantuan rooster presiding over several dogs, an elephant, a tabby cat, Santa Claus, birds and teacups. On a table beside the television set, a few impressive trophies were mixed in with framed family photographs.

I asked James about the trophies, and about the photograph of him displayed on one wall, in U.S. Navy blues, a white sailor cap. He told me, modestly, that he had played basketball for Beauregard High, and enlisted in the Navy after he graduated. He had gotten a medical discharge from the Navy because he'd been diagnosed as having leukemia. He had had to go to Seattle, Washington, for a bone marrow transplant at the VA Hospital there. Eileen and her daughter, Julia, had gone to Seattle with James, moving into the VA Hospital apartment annex for visiting family members. Eileen told us how nice everyone was out there. James nodded in agreement. "Yes," he said, "they were good to us out there."

Eileen touched the heart-shaped locket at her throat, shifting her legs in the armchair. She couldn't get over how nasty that apartment was, food on the floor, roaches everywhere. She'd stayed up until 1 A.M. the night she moved in, cleaning up the place. But the Lord had blessed them, for the transplant had been successful. And the people—*peoples* she actually said—were so nice to them. She had the Lord to thank for that.

Leaving, we talked with James outside the house. The boat he went fishing in was parked in the back yard. He told us he did a lot of tournament fishing, and had also helped put on a casting demonstration for deprived kids, in Montgomery. His father had taken him fishing when he was a boy. Eileen had gotten that across to us, how James loved fishing. James wasn't over his illness, so he didn't have that much stamina. But fishing, that was something he was able to do. James also told us about a shorter way to get to Eileen's place from Auburn. We could get there in half the time it had taken us using Lee 51.

ON MY SECOND VISIT, I followed James's directions, Lee 412 to the Lazy Bee, then a right on Lee 54. I passed a road leading to sequestered country houses for people who made their money in Auburn but preferred to reside in the country. The sign at the entrance read SERENITY. At Lee 27 there was another sign with an arrow—PINE BREEZE TRAILER RANCH. Follow the arrow northeast, I thought, and you might get lucky and see some trailers going this way. The road was thickly hedged in with pines until, suddenly, there was #6221, the familiar house set back from the road, its sun-drenched, sand-packed drive awaiting me. I made a left turn, pulled on in, turned the motor off, and got out of the car.

Augustine was nowhere to be seen, so I went up to the front door and knocked. I heard Eileen humming a spiritual, and then she was opening the door for me, welcoming me with a broad smile. An air conditioner, a 110 window unit, was running (Linda had been mistaken about the lack of air conditioning). Eileen was wearing the same dress she had worn before, and the heart-shaped locket was on its thin gold chain. For the first time I noticed she was wearing canvas shoes, very flimsy, more like house slippers, with a shiny green palm tree on each instep.

We didn't stay long with Cassie Binton. Cassie thought Eileen had been to church, she thought it was Sunday, not Tuesday. Her mind, Eileen told me on our way back to the living room, hadn't been right for years, long before she'd gotten the cancer last November. When Cassie's sister Susie Mae died, Cassie had started hiding things in the house. She needed to be cooking all the time, and was always turning on the gas burners. Eileen couldn't leave Cassie alone for a minute.

Once we were back in the living room, Eileen motioned for me to take the rocker across from the sofa. Eileen sat down in the armchair across from me. She picked up a coffee mug on the end table beside her chair. She took a sip of coffee, replacing the mug on the end table. After I settled into the rocker, I asked Eileen what she did for a living. She told me she had worked in housekeeping, at East Alabama Medical Center for fifteen years. After that she had worked at the hospital laundry for eleven years. She said that the man who managed the hospital (she couldn't recollect his name) didn't like black folks. He was friendly with the white folks but he never spoke to the black folks who worked there.

I had to ask her, "Wouldn't he have had to speak to a black nurse, or someone in administration who was black?" She looked at me dubiously, then peremptorily replied, "I tell you he hates black folks."

It wasn't long before she was talking my arm off. And I was listening intently. One thing that came through to me was her need for someone to listen to her. I was caught up in the way her life had gone, what she hated and what she felt was right. She had done what she had to do, and she didn't want, or expect, any free rides. She had worked hard and had earned everything she'd gotten.

Some people, she went on, are just lucky. They get things free somehow. But there was this old woman she knew without anything, no water, not even an electric fan, and it got so hot she had to go out on the porch at night because she couldn't stand it inside. And finally someone saw her sitting out on her porch and they brought her a fan. Can you imagine that, having to sit out on your porch at night? But others, they took advantage. She knew someone who even got his electricity free, not just food stamps and welfare. Eileen didn't want anything handed to her. Some people would do anything to get something for nothing. She knew these black folks who wanted a new car so bad they sat out in one all night. The dealer would give you the car if you sat in it for twenty-four hours, she said, and that meant you couldn't get out of the car, you had to eat and sleep right there. She wouldn't do that, even if they gave her the car. She'd rather earn the money for a car.

Taking another sip of coffee, Eileen abruptly changed the subject. She launched into what drugs were doing to black kids. It was the drugs for her. People were selling the drugs right here on this road till the "po-lice" came and broke it up. And marijuana beds were all over. When you saw a low-flying airplane, you knew the po-lice were looking for marijuana. "And these kids killing themselves with guns, and the men in jail in their air-conditioned cells just laying around watchin' TV, I say put 'em to work." She had some bad things to say about drug dealing in Tuskegee, fifteen miles down Highway 129 from Auburn. Tuskegee had been a good place to live in once, but now the drugs were everywhere and the po-lice, they looked the other way. She had gone to live there with her husband—that was before they were separated—and he'd gotten into dealing in drugs and that just did it for her. She told him she didn't want him in the house anymore. So he cleared out; he moved to Birmingham. She moved back here to be with her father.

She had a nephew, Roy—such a sweet boy he was. Little Roy was living with his grandmama then. His mama had gone off somewhere and was sending the grandmama money to take care of Roy, but the grandmama she didn't care for Roy. She kept the money and spent it on herself. So Roy, he didn't have anything, no one to raise him and nowhere to go. Roy started hanging around with this gang of older boys that sold drugs. He wasn't doing the

drugs himself, but he was with the ones who did. They tried to
hold up the insurance man—he'd be running the debit, I figured,
collecting premiums in cash on burial policies—but the police
caught them and they were sent to prison.

I asked Eileen if Roy was still in prison. She said he was, but
that might have saved his life, she said, shifting her body in the
armchair, smoothing her tight dress out below her big knees. "I
thank the Lord he is in prison because otherwise he'd be dead
now," she said.

PARKING MY CAR in the driveway, I saw James out in the back of
the house. I thought of going around to the kitchen door, in order
to ask James where the dog was, the dog I'd heard about but so
far hadn't encountered. What if Augustine were an apocryphal
dog, spoken of but never showing up? Without taking note of
my presence, James disappeared through the back door. The
sun-baked porch chairs to the left of the front steps kept their
rigid alignment.

I heard Eileen hymn-humming from inside the house. Then she
was greeting me at the front door. She was wearing a low-necked
sleeveless dress, an inky blue, flower-splotched dress, its vermilion
petaled, green-leafy flowers floating in turquoise amoeba flecked
ponds. She was wearing the palm tree slippers. Her hair seemed
darker today. As she settled herself in her armchair, I realized she
might be wanting to show me she could still fit into this dress. I sat
down in the rocker. From somewhere down the hall, James flitted
into the kitchen. With a scratched-out smile, he said in passing,
"I'm mowing the lawn." I didn't hear him close the back door.

Eileen offered to turn on the air conditioner. I realized that
would run up her power bill, so I said I was all right without it.
The television set stayed on while we talked, which made it hard
to make out what Eileen was saying sometimes. Yet the gist of

her talk was pretty clear to me. Raising kids, using the switch on them. No you don't say next time I'll whip you. And more on the drugs, on the killings. And on earning what you got, being able to do without. Eileen pulled a handkerchief out from below her neckline and patted her forehead. She said she could do without a TV. She spread the handkerchief out in her lap. I heard the power mower putt-putting outside. This white lady down the road, Mrs. Moberly, she was telling Eileen she'd wished she didn't have a TV. You won't like it after you've had it awhile. And what if Eileen got one of those telephones where you could see who you were talking to. Her forehead wrinkling above raised eyebrows, Eileen imitated Mrs. Moberly—"and what if you were in the bathtub Eileen and someone called you while you were there, what would you do then?"

"I told Mrs. Moberly I didn't know what I would do. But you won't catch me with one of them telephones."

We had a good laugh, then fell silent. As if she felt she had verged on immodesty, Eileen looked at the figurines in the cabinet mounted over the sofa on one wall, the rooster, the dogs, the elephant. I looked at the crocheted message on another wall, GOOD DEEDS LIVE LONG. The lawn mower droned in the front yard.

Pretty soon, two black women came in through the kitchen. They said hello and trooped back to the bedroom. They were the women here to bathe Cassie. They bathed Cassie on weekdays; Eileen had to bathe Cassie on weekends. That was a hard job for one person to do. Eileen told me she had been up with Cassie last night until three or four in the morning. What were you having to do? I asked her hesitantly, but she didn't mind telling me. What kept her up was the choking; she had to put the suction tube down Cassie's throat. Suck the mucus up, she was telling me. I asked her how Cassie was fed and she said through this tube in her stomach. She fed Cassie milk through the tube.

It wasn't long before Cassie was bathed and dressed, and once the women were on their way, I asked Eileen if we could see her now. Yes, we can go on back now, Eileen said, pushing her left foot into a canvas slipper.

Cassie wore a light blue cotton nightgown. Her thin arms were outside the blanket, her long-fingered, mahogany-hued hands lying still. Her breathing was labored, rasping. I said, "I'm sorry you're feeling bad." I touched one limp hand, avoiding looking at the wall with the paint peeling off. "It's a nice day, not that hot," I said.

Cassie looked up at me. It was as if she were allowing me to look down at her as long as I liked.

Squatting between the two beds was an ugly robotic machine with an aluminum boxlike base, surmounted by a glass bulb containing a yellowish liquid. A plastic tube slithered out of its base, crawled up the side of the bed and disappeared under Cassie's blanket, the same tube emerging from beneath the bed, snaking over to the glass bulb, rearing up to fasten its mouth on a kind of spigot in the glass bulb. I asked Eileen what this tube was for, without anticipating what Eileen would do next. Eileen went to Cassie, flipped the blanket down to show me the pouch on Cassie's stomach. "That's where the tube goes in," Eileen said, raising the blanket again. "That's where I feed her the milk. That tube on the floor is for her discharges." I looked at Cassie's liquid waste pooling in the bulb. Her body was a living conduit for food and waste.

Cassie went on gazing upward.

BEFORE I MADE MY NEXT VISIT, I telephoned Eileen and asked if I could bring her a gift—a framed print that had once belonged to an eccentric artist friend, Dorothy Doaty. Dorothy was moving to Gulf Breeze, Florida, with her multitudinous paintings and drawings and six overfed and overcoddled cats. She was trying to dispose of the print, along with other picturesque items she didn't have room for in her newly rented house. So I asked her if I could have it, thinking Eileen might accept it from me. We could put it up on the bedroom wall.

The print was from the collection of Robert Forbes; it read at the bottom, "Gardener at Kensington Gardens, 1730," and above, that in upper case—DECEMBER. Stalks, leaves and flowers, intertwined stems, snippets of anemic color jammed into a single stone vase, the botanical riches of December exfoliated in profusion, numbered from one to thirty and identified in the legend below. For instance, 3, Panzies or Hearts Ease, 14, Winter White Primrose, 27, Scarlet Geraniums. Painted on the vase was a recumbent male and female nude, and a hovering cupid.

Once I had Eileen on the telephone, I mentioned the picture in an offhand way. "I can bring it on out today, Eileen, if you'd really like to have it."

"Yes, I would like that," Eileen said, with measured formality.

It was early in October. The first hint of autumn was in the air. Driving out, I saw clumps of goldenrod on each side of the road, Black Eyed Susans, a few shreds of summer's Queen Anne's Lace. Pulling into the congenial, familiar drive, I looked for Augustine. No sign of him. He must be on the other side of the road, somewhere in the woods. But what was this pale yellow fire hydrant to my left, close to the road, upthrusting? Why hadn't I noticed that before? Would Augustine come bounding out of the woods, cock a leg up, spatter the hydrant. I didn't ask Eileen what the hydrant was doing in her front yard, but I did inquire after Augustine. Eileen told me the dog spent his days in the woods. In the evening, she fed him leftovers at the back door, and brother

Tim fed him dog food. Augustine was a no-account hound dog, not good for hunting or much else, she said. Whatever he was, I was thinking I would never meet up with him. And that was all right with me.

Eileen was wearing the light blue dress she had worn on the day I met her. A large safety pin hooked up buttons that threatened to pop loose any second. I didn't speculate on the safety pin, being occupied with presenting Cassie's picture to her. She was taken with it. Right away I saw that it was special for her.

"Why it's a boaoh—kay," she drawled out, with a broad smile.

"That's right," I replied, "a December bouquet."

I went on to explain what the picture was doing, how the numbered flowers and plants matched the identifications, and showed her the inscription below. "From the Collection of Robert Forbes, Gardener at Kensington," I read out to her, "1730," and Eileen mmmed and ahhhed over how long ago that was.

We went on back to the bedroom. Cassie was asleep, breathing stertorously through fluttering lips, her hands folded over her lavender nightgown, a little crone-doll with twin gray plaits poking out from her ears like antennae. She'd been awake last night coughing a lot. Eileen had to give her some milk through the PEG tube issuing from the robotic machine; that helped sometimes, she told me. Cassie looked pleased and comfortable, I thought, as if she were dreaming sweet dreams. The question nipped away in my brain: what would dreaming be like if you were terminal, sick unto death but not dying yet, before the time came to babble of green fields, cross over the river, give up the ghost?

We decided to hang the picture between the door and Eileen's cluttered vanity. The picture lacked eye hooks spanned by a wire; instead it had to hang from a crevice in the frame. That might be dangerous if we hung this picture on Cassie's wall. Eileen quickly reassured me by saying Cassie could see it from across the room. I couldn't find a stud in that section of wall, so I had to knock a nail through the plaster. I inserted one of the Phillips screws Eileen brought me, tipped the frame over the depressed screw. The picture stayed up, so we left it there. Cassie was still sleeping when we left.

Once again we were sitting across from each other. I was settled in the familiar rocker. Eileen didn't have the television on, so the listening was easier today. And I got some words in edgewise, asked some questions, learned some things.

I learned a good deal about Eileen's father, Johnny Hooper. He was on dialysis in his later years. He had to go into the hospital daily. The night he died (he was ninety-one) he refused to go for the treatment. He told Eileen he wouldn't be coming back, and she told him he had to go, she didn't know how to do dialysis here. He did go, brother Tim took him, and then the hospital called. They had moved Mr. Hooper into ICU. Eileen was told her father was going fast, she should get on over to the hospital. She said she knew he'd be gone when she got there so she didn't go, she couldn't.

Johnny Hooper had had diabetes for years and had lost both his legs. He was a good man who had led a hard life. He had this house built on the land owned by Eileen's grandfather. Her grandfather had bought the land from a white man, Mr. Moberly, who owned a lot of land up and down the road. But before her father moved here, they had lived three miles outside Opelika. Her father worked the graveyard shift at Pepperell Mill, from eleven to seven, five nights a week, and on Saturday he worked cutting meat at Story's Grocery Store afternoons and nights. Every weeknight at seven he'd walk three miles to a friend's place near the mill, take a nap, then go to work. He'd walk back at seven in the morning and farm all day. "I used to say, 'Daddy you can't do no farm work and keep on at the mill.' But he told me he reckoned he could do that." Later on, after they had this house built, Johnny Hooper walked to Pepperell Mill every day, eight miles each way.

Eileen moved back into this house with her father later on. She had been living in Tuskegee with her husband, but when she found out he was dealing in drugs, she left him and took her children with her. She had gotten the housekeeping job at the hospital (I didn't tell her she had told me that). She had been offered a job as a nurse's aide, but she had turned it down because she couldn't stand cleaning sick people up. "You'd be surprised how filthy they can be," she said. She had had to clean up her daddy, and then Cassie's sister, Susie Mae, and now she was cleaning up Cassie since the Hospice bathers didn't come on weekends.

I prepared myself to hear a litany of privations. Instead Eileen veered off to her son, James Foote, his bone marrow transplant, how he needed to take care of himself. At some point in the conversation, I told Eileen that my sister-in-law had been a bone marrow transplant donor once. Eileen quickly brought the conversation back to her family; she said her daughter, Julia, had been the donor for James. Eileen had known anonymous donors were available, but Julia had done the transplant just fine, and Eileen had done the blood transfusion.

We reached a high point in her new narrative. The good Lord had helped her that time, she said. Julia had a certain type of sensitive skin. There was no way to get the tape off without pulling Julia's skin off with it. The tape was driving poor Julia wild. No one Eileen asked for help knew what to do, not the doctors, "no one," she told me, "but the good Lord, He told me what to do." Eileen drew her shoulders back a little, her hands resting lightly on the arms of the chair, and spoke as if God were talking: "You go to the store and get Crisco, Eileen. You slap the Crisco on

Julia's bed sheet and you make her lie on it all night." So Eileen did that, slapped Crisco on the sheet and made Julia lie down on it all night. The next morning the tape came right off. "Right off, like the good Lord told me it would."

Before I left I asked to see Cassie again. Cassie was awake, so Eileen pointed out the picture to her. "That's a boah-kay. Isn't it pretty?" Cassie saw it, but she was still groggy from sleep. Her lips were working, almost inaudible muttered words trickling out.

I went up to Cassie and picked her left hand up from its place on the lavender nightgown. Eileen rearranged the sheet so Cassie's flat chest was decently covered. Cassie had her other hand on her belly, where the PEG tube was inserted, embedded in tape. I held Cassie's hand a little while longer. I said I hoped she liked the picture. Then I said I had to be going but I'd be back to see her next week. Something astonishing happened then. A rush of pleasure swept over Cassie's face.

"Do that," she said, in a high, perky voice.

DRIVING BACK ON LEE 54, I saw two men cutting a broad swathe on the opposite side of the road, their clacking mowers spaced one behind the other. I breathed in the smell of newly mown grass. A little later, before stopping off at the Lazy Bee to use the men's room and pick up a Diet Coke, I sat in my car and read the sign on the window.

Harry Lazenby
Lee County Rd 54 . . . 412.
7 AM–9 PM
In case of emergency
Call 205 745 6621.

In case of emergency.

Eileen's father had gotten off work at 7 A.M. He might have taken this road on his long walk home, passed the Lazy Bee, kept on going.

5

In Search of J. R. R. Tolkien

O N A FRIDAY AFTERNOON in early October, I had a scrawled-over legal pad propped up on the dining room table, what I'd written the day before at Burger King, a cup of instant decaf, a bowl of hard candy to rev me up for the rewriting process. Through the French doors, beyond the screened-in back porch, two cardinals, a male and a female, were at the feeding tray to the bird feeder hanging from a branch of a cottonwood tree out back. A squirrel was edging close to the feeder; I was about to shoo off the squirrel when the telephone rang. It was Linda Merritt.

Linda wanted to know if I would be willing to see another patient while I was seeing Cassie Binton. I asked her whom she had in mind. A retired chemistry professor, Larry Beckwith, she said quietly—she was being very low keyed about this assignment—Larry had taught at Tuskegee Institute. He and his wife and son lived in Auburn, on South Gay Street. "I thought Larry might appreciate having you read something to him."

I hesitated a moment, on the verge of asking Linda if I could have a day or two to think about it. Seeing two patients instead of one would take away from my writing time.

"I really think Larry would like having you as a volunteer."

Two finches joined the cardinals. The note of urgency in Linda's voice impelled me not to wait to make a commitment.

"All right. I'll do it," I said. "Actually, I can start next week. Would mornings be better or afternoons?"

"Sometime in the morning, I'm thinking. Larry's wife Catherine teaches in the morning. At Tuskegee Institute. She tells me Larry's son would be there two mornings a week, but the other three he has to go to East Alabama Medical Center for dialysis. So you would be a help to her."

"Would Wednesday morning be all right?"

"I'll have to check and see. I'll call Catherine tonight, and get back to you."

"Any morning would be okay. Just let me know when."

Once Linda was off the line, two finches joined the cardinals at the feeding trough. The male finch let the female eat first. That is chivalry, I said to myself. I got up and went outside and tossed a beat-up tennis ball at the squirrel, who scurried to safety in the cottonwood's topmost branches. Pine straw silted the back yard, the hint of a chill in the air. Larry Beckwith, Catherine Beckwith. Cassie Binton, Eileen Foote. I would be seeing both patients, both caregivers. What did Larry Beckwith and Cassie Binton have in common? Nothing much. From the standpoint of race, gender, education, even age, they were as different as night and day. And the same was true for the family members. In a sense, I would be acting in different plays, on different stages, suiting, as Hamlet put it, the action to the word. And on a third stage, my own back yard, I watched the male finch take his turn at the trough. I would return to a word processor, a Mac Plus, peer at almost indecipherable words purporting to represent actual life, type them onto a screen, nudge one here, delete several there. I would become the actor as writer, with the help of this computer impervious to pain, temporarily exempt from death, acting on another stage, without an audience. Where male finches were unaccountably chivalrous, at least for me. Or was that true of all Southern finches?

A grackle bore down on the feeder, scattering finches and cardinals, reminding me that living was more than mere acting. I wondered what I could do to make Larry Beckwith's life easier.

As IT TURNED OUT, we would be making our first visit on Thursday morning, a little before ten A.M. As she had before, Linda Merritt would drive me to the patient's home, and when we got there, she would introduce me, and with her customary tact make it easier for Larry and me to make contact.

I showed up at Linda's office at nine-thirty. Before we left, I read over Larry's Hospice data sheet:

    Patient: Dr. Larry Beckwith (Ph.D.)

    Date of Referral : 8/21/98

    Date of Admission: 9/2/98

    Spouse or Significant Other: Dr. Katherine Beckwith

    Address : 550 South Gay Street Auburn Ala 36830

    Telephone : (334) 887 9692

    Date of Birth: 10/14/40

    Race: White

    Age: 57

    Diagnosis: Metastatic colon cancer

    Caregivers :Katherine Beckwith (wife), Jason Beckwith (son)

    Church: St. Andrew's Episcopal Tuskegee

    Description of present status: wt. 152, ht. 5' 7"

    Awake but lethargic, ambulatory in home. Difficulty completing thought processes. Color jaundiced. Abdomen very large, liver edge easily palpable, c/o pain in LVQ nausea slightly improved. Has occasional diarrhea. Noticeably weaker and less alert . . . wishes palliative care.

Living arrangements: Lives with wife and son in large home, son is chronically ill.

Level of activity: Ambulatory

Limitations imposed by illness: Weak, nauseated

Recreation/Hobbies/Occupation: chemistry Professor at Tuskegee University; Music: trumpet, piano, vocal baritone

We hadn't far to go this time, for the Beckwiths lived on South Gay Street, in an older section of Auburn. Across the street was Lipscomb Park, one of many small parks situated in older Auburn neighborhoods. Three horseshoe curved stone benches, two outdoor grills, a picnic table, a rudimentary jungle jim, that was about the extent of this park, no swings or teeter-totters, no sliding board.

The park blended into the neighborhood, the quiet, low-profiled ranch houses, the broad front yards strewn with pine-straw. Election placards had sprouted all over town, so I wasn't surprised to see four stilted excrescences sprouting from the front yard of the Beckwiths' neighbors to the north, their bold primary colors standing out in the lambent afternoon light.

The house itself was weathered brick. It had a carport with enough room to accommodate one car, a spiffy dark blue Mazda Miata. A fire-engine red Trans-Am was parked catty-cornered in the front yard.

Linda and I went to the front door first, faced with its scrollwork window set in formidable looking oak, the heavy iron knocker that challenged one of us to knock. Linda stepped up and did the knocking. Nobody answered, so we decided we'd try the kitchen door. The direct way to the carport was a walkway between the house and a box hedge, but the walkway was blocked by stacks of books, bound dark blue volumes of *The Journal of the American Chemical Society,* protected by the overhanging roof. We had to work our way around the box hedge, scuffing pine straw, to get to the carport.

Linda rapped her knuckles on the glass-sectioned kitchen door, perhaps a little too loud, but then she hadn't been heard at the front door. It wasn't long before Larry Beckwith came shuffling through the kitchen. He stopped at the door and peered out at us, as if at visitors he might not want to admit, and then the door opened and Linda was saying we were a little late, would it be all right if we stayed a little while? "Certainly, I was expecting you," Larry Beckwith said, in a low voice, almost a whisper.

Larry closed the kitchen door as soon as we were inside the sunlit kitchen. He was wearing a NIKE-emblazoned T-shirt too tight for his knobby shoulders, lightweight burgundy polyester jogging pants, natty tan socks, snug-fitting cordovan loafers. He had a light brown mustache curling up a little at each end, graying hair. His transition lenses seemed to be adjusting to the gloom beyond the kitchen, as he led us on to the living room. By letting us in he could shut the outside world out, all the worrisome things he wasn't concerned with now, his two dogs in the fenced-in back yard, the still unraked pine straw, the bound volumes behind the box hedge. The necessary introducing—Larry shook my hand with some firmness—that too behind him. We moved through this rambling, lived-in house and found a seat on the sofa. Larry sat down in a chair in front of the picture window and the glass doors to the patio. He crossed his legs, his back to the sunlight streaming in through the window.

Linda sat down on a sofa at a right angle to Larry's chair, and I sat down beside her. A clock was ticking on the mantel above the fireplace, punctuating the silence that had taken over the sick man's darkened living room. It was Larry who spoke first. He asked us if he could get us something to drink.

"I guess not," Linda said politely. I mumbled, "No thanks."

The clock ticked on, the silence extending between us. Suddenly, Larry's black and white cat jumped up on the coffee table. Lifting his tail, the cat meowed vociferously. Larry smiled. "That's Wiley's way of telling me he wants out." He moved a little in his chair. "If you'll excuse me a moment, I'll let him out."

"No, let me do it," I said hastily. I got up from the sofa. Wiley waited for me on the coffee table. His pupils narrowing to slits, he let out an earsplitting meow.

Larry got to his feet. "Thanks for offering, but I'll have to do it."

Once Larry was back from the kitchen, settled in the armchair again, he asked Linda how long she had been with Hospice. After she filled him in on her career, he asked me how long I had been a volunteer. I said I'd gotten started last May. I went on to say I'd been a college professor at Auburn University for thirty-four years, that I had retired from teaching in 1994. I brought up a friend, Ruth Morehouse, who had retired from Tuskegee Institute—she had taught in the art department—and it turned out Larry knew her. He asked me how Ruth was doing, and I said she was painting, traveling a lot with her husband, doing all right.

The conversation trailed off, then picked up again. Larry talked about his own retirement as if it had little to do with his illness. One problem he had had was what to do with his books, which were piling up all over the house. Yes, I had noticed books stacked outside, behind the box hedge. Without offense (for none had been meant) he replied in his quiet voice, "Well, I don't really have any need for them. The chemistry journals are on microfiche now. But since I don't know what to do with them, they'll have to stay out there for awhile."

I told him that since I had retired I'd had to move books out from my office at school. I didn't have enough bookcases at home for all of them, so I had to store a lot of books in the attic. Then I asked him how long he'd been at Tuskegee Institute. He said he started in 1997. "No that's obviously not right. It was in 1967."

We didn't talk that long. Linda asked Larry if he was interested in having me read to him. He nodded his head. That would be all right, he said. I asked him if he had any preferences. He said he was interested in religious literature, but he would leave the choice up to me.

"I might not be that good a listener. It's difficult for me to stay focused."

"We'll try it and see what happens," I said.

"That will be fine," Larry said.

Another pause notched by the ticking clock. Larry's face clouded over.

"Could you come back the week after next? My sister is coming to visit next week."

"The week after next is fine with me."

Linda asked Larry where his sister was from. From Indiana, Pennsylvania, Larry said. Linda latched on conversationally to Indiana, Pennsylvania. "That's a tough one," she said, "that's like who's on first." Who's on what? I was unable to see much of a connection between Abbott and Costello and Indiana, Pennsylvania. Smoothing her skirt out, Linda went on to say Hospice would send someone over to rake the yard before his sister arrived next week. Larry said his son Jason usually raked the yard, but Jason hadn't gotten to it yet. It would be fine if someone from Hospice raked the yard. In fact he didn't realize Hospice did all these things.

"Oh yes," Linda said glancing at me, "we can do a lot of things. We can send a volunteer to cut your hair too."

"Well that would be nice, but I wouldn't ask you to do that."

"Don't ask me," I said, half-jocularly, "I'm not much good at cutting hair."

Larry said, "I can understand that."

Our eyes met. I realized we had a rapport, a mutual trust.

Then the clock was ticking, sunlight streaming in through the picture window. Larry Beckwith crossed his legs.

ANOTHER SUNNY DAY, the sky fluffed with slow-moving cumuli, a light breeze stirring the leaves of the big-branched elm behind the low-slung house. The pine straw hadn't been raked up after all. Only one patch of shiny zoysia showed, where the Trans-Am had been parked two weeks ago. I shuffled on up the driveway into the carport, passing blue-backed volumes of *The Journal of the American Chemical Society* stacked behind the box hedge. Larry's blue Miata was parked a little away from the kitchen door. I shifted the paperback in my right hand to my left hand before I knocked, pausing to take in the pyracantha bushes along the other side of the carport, their berries just getting their first blush. I hadn't long to wait before Larry came to the door. He unlocked it before he opened it.

He was wearing the burgundy polyester jogging pants, the Nike T-shirt, cordovan house slippers, tan socks. We shook hands in the kitchen, and then I followed him into the living room. He went straight to the sofa. I took the armchair, my back to the picture window. Larry lay down on the sofa, his head pillowed on one armrest, a lightweight blanket covering his legs. The clock on the mantel was ticking. Wiley the cat was nowhere to be seen, and Jason too wouldn't be with us. This was one of the days Jason had dialysis.

I didn't know how to begin. Finally— "It's a nice day we're having, don't you think?"

"Yes, it's a beautiful day," Larry said quietly.

I kept a paperback volume of *The Hobbit* closed while we continued our sporadic, halting conversation. He had enjoyed seeing his sister, he said. It had been a good visit. Since he'd grown up in Pennsylvania, I mentioned growing up in Kokomo, Indiana, for that was something of a coincidence, how Indiana figured in both of our lives. He'd grown up on a dairy farm in northwest Pennsylvania, not in Indiana, Pennsylvania. That was where his sister lived now. He didn't tell me the name of the town, waiting for what I had to say next. I said a little more about Kokomo. Kokomo, I went on, is known as the city of firsts; that's inscribed on the city limits sign—two firsts were the Haines automobile and, in the city park, the world's largest stuffed moose. Larry's smile came back, but he was having trouble maintaining it. I realized I had come here to read, not talk.

That morning I had made a final choice, after mulling over what to read to Larry the night before. On my first visit, with Linda Merritt, Larry had expressed a preference for religious literature. I wasn't sure what Larry meant by religious literature? *Pilgrim's Progress?* A novel from a Christian perspective? A story by Nathaniel Hawthorne? I considered reading "Young Goodman Brown." Then there was devotional poetry, Gerard Manley Hopkins, George Herbert, T. S. Eliot. Or I might stay away from religious literature; after all, Larry had said the choice was mine. I might read some Chekhov, something not too long, like "Misery" or "The Darling"? I was still in a quandary when I went to bed that night. In a rush the next morning to be on my way, I took one last tour of my bookshelves. One book seemed to leap out at my hand. Why not J. R. R. Tolkien, why not *The Hobbit?*

The Hobbit was hopeful, not nihilistic or existentialist. Moreover, *The Hobbit* would be easy for Larry to follow, and one could argue, it had religious implications. Once I had the paperback out of the shelf, I remembered the Hospice meeting I'd gone to last week, in which we talked about reading children's stories, something to evoke childhood, a sense of wonderment. But Larry Beckwith was far from being a child; he knew where he was, what he had to face; he might not care to be patronized. Still, *The Hobbit* seemed the right choice. With Larry lying down on the sofa, trying to muster up what little energy he had to converse with me, I knew I could not turn back; I was here to read to him, and read to him I must. The paperback Tolkien was in my left hand, waiting to be opened. So when our talked lapsed into silence—I was hoping Wiley would show up and give me a reprieve, but he didn't—I came out with it:

"Would you like to have me read *The Hobbit?* It's a fantasy novel by J. R. R. Tolkien. In *The Hobbit,* and in his great trilogy, *The Lord of the Rings,* he takes some of the material you find in epic and saga, and puts it into a new context." Larry pulled the blanket up over his legs. I went on, half apologetically. "The Hobbit may be just an entertaining fantasy, but we can try it, see how it goes."

Larry's smile was back, and his eyes were bright. "Okay. Let's try it," he said.

I opened the book, glad to be underway, intoning, "Chapter One, 'An Unexpected Party.'"

> In a hole in the ground there lived a hobbit. Not a nasty, dirty, wet hole, filled with the ends of worms and an oozy smell, nor yet a dry, bare, sandy hole with nothing to sit down on or to eat; it was a hobbit-hole and that means comfortable.

IN LARRY'S COMFORTABLE living room—no not nasty and wet or sandy and bare—I heard the sound of my voice, the clock ticking whenever I paused. I kept my eyes on the opening pages, inflecting my voice as I read, trying to capture Bilbo's tightlipped British conventionality—"We don't want any adventures here, thank you. You might try over the hill or over the Water"—or Gandalf's Trevor-Howard-like well-bred bossiness—"Put us on a few eggs, there's a good fellow," and the dwarves—well, think of Disney's dwarves, picturesque little guys; just keep them clamorous and shrill.

Time was passing as I read words on a page, words meant for childlike grown-ups or, in the United States in the sixties, flower children on LSD, with a low threshold of disbelief. Occasionally, my eyes left the page, wondered off to Larry stretched out on the sofa, his head turned away, one hand flat on one side of his face, as if he were listening to classical music. He might be listening to me or resting. He would glance over at me during a long pause, and let me know I should keep on reading. I shifted the paperback from hand to hand, crossed my legs, extended them out on the carpet, savoring the leathery comfort of the armchair. It was all right for me to be here in another man's house reading Chapter I of *The Hobbit*.

When the dwarves sang out their tale of stolen gold, I did a kind of chanting replication of what the dwarves might sound like.

> The bells were ringing in the dale
> And men looked up with faces pale
> The dragon's ire more fierce than fire
> Laid low their towers and houses frail.

With his head propped up on his hand, Larry listened intently to the song.

It is established early in Chapter I that Bilbo Baggins had a hell-raising, adventure-seeking grandfather Took, on his mother's side, through whom Bilbo had gotten "something that only waited to come out." Soon after the dwarves finally finish their song (it runs ten stanzas), Bilbo has a sudden urge to go on an adventure himself. "Something Tookish woke up inside him, and he wished to go see the great mountains, and hear the pine-trees and the waterfalls, and explore the caves, and wear a sword instead of a walking stick." But soon Bilbo's imagination gets the better of his newly discovered derring-do. He sees a flame leap up, outside the window—or it could be someone lighting up a wood fire—and terrified of plundering dragons outside, he shudders, and very soon he is cautious, comfortable Mr. Baggins again.

I stopped to make a comment. "I guess his Baggins side wants to play it safe, even though he does have this Took side that wants, maybe needs, to have adventures."

Larry smiled. "Yes, I see that," he said.

I shifted the paperback, stretched my legs. Rearranging the blanket, Larry shifted his legs on the sofa. Both of us were getting comfortable, pulled into a cozy Tolkienian hobbithood, which was sustained for awhile in my reading, the clock ticking, autumn sunlight outside the window.

After I finished the first chapter, I said that might be enough for today. I started talking about the symbolism of the dragon—in Tolkien's book a worm named Smaug—and the treasure Smaug is guarding, in terms of Carl Jung and Eric Neumann, as elements of the collective unconscious manifested in myth and dream as well as in heroic saga. The treasure is one form of the Jungian anima, as treasure a displacement of the maiden-bride for the male, and the dragon is the destructive mother archetype. I also touched on Joseph Campbell's hero with a thousand faces, asserting that Bilbo Baggins, a middle-class nonviolent man, is still capable, Tolkien is saying, of slaying a dragon. Larry Beckwith listened intently, and went on to say yes, that might be so. But I'm not sure he really thought it was so.

Before I left I asked Larry if he wanted me to read a little poetry next time. I still had Hopkins and Eliot in mind if Tolkien turned out to be too whimsical. Larry said he wasn't much on poetry, in a matter of fact, non-apologetic way. He said he hadn't really read much poetry.

I closed up the book but stayed in my chair. "All right, we'll keep on with *The Hobbit*, if that's all right with you."

"That will be all right with me."

It was time to leave the leathery comfort of the armchair. On my feet, I said to Larry I could find my own way out, no need for him to get up. I'd be back about this time next week.

"Next week. That will be fine," Larry said.

For a moment I hovered over the sofa. Without raising his head, Larry raised his right hand and clasped my right hand.

The next time I came, around noon on October 20, there was a white sedan parked in front of the Miata. Jason's Trans-Am was occupying its diagonal slot in the front yard. I had brought one of my published short stories along with me as a last minute alternative to reading on in *The Hobbit*. Just before I got out of my car, I considered leaving the story behind, even though it was relatively easy to follow. No, why not take it with me, in case my reading of *The Hobbit* fell flat.

The story is entitled "Pagoda." It appeared in an obscure literary review "for emerging writers over sixty." A middle-aged man with a bad heart—he might go any moment—finds himself watching a bird feeder in his back yard. He's out of a job, but since he has an independent income, he can pretend to bide his time while he sends out resumes that he knows will never be considered. His wife is trying to be there for him, but she is also attracted to a muscular young handy man. She keeps finding jobs for him to do in the house and yard—he will even build a new boat dock before the story is over. The main character finally accepts his mortality and the eventual loss of his wife; he even plays Ping-Pong (he loses consistently) with the handyman. In the course of the story, his view of the bird feeder—a three-tiered structure with overhanging roofs bearing a resemblance to a Chinese pagoda—shifts from obsessive-compulsive scrutiny to something akin to Zen-like illumination. Now that it doesn't matter when he dies, he can see the feeder differently. "I see it as an image, a metaphor. It's a temple, a kind of pagoda, in a garden where there are exotic birds. . . .It isn't literally a pagoda, but it could be where pagodas are found."

I had "Pagoda" with me when I knocked on the kitchen door, but once inside, shaking hands with Larry's wife Katherine, I knew I wouldn't read this story. A slender, loose-jointed woman with short black hair, wearing glasses, still attractive, wearing slacks and a man's white shirt, which she hadn't tucked in, Katherine Beckwith greeted me pleasantly, yet with a reserve that enforced my awareness of this family's belief in privacy. As I followed her to the living room, I felt like an intruder, one witnessing things he wasn't meant to see. In this case, balloons in the living room, three balloons, red, blue, and silver, floating high over the mantel to which they were tethered, "Happy Birthday" inscribed on each festive balloon.

Larry was lying on the sofa, the blanket pulled up above his knees. He wasn't wearing the Nike T-shirt or the burgundy pants; today he wore a motley bathrobe and pajamas. He apologized for not getting up. I had taken my seat in the armchair. Katherine was standing by Larry, holding his hand in hers. Yes, his birthday party took place yesterday, on October fourteenth. Mine was coming up on October sixteenth. That wasn't so bad, we were both Libras, and the balloons, still aloft, floating cheerily as balloons invariably must, might also be celebrating our Librahood.

We made small talk for a little while, and then the reading of *The Hobbit* came up. Raising his head, Larry told me he might go to sleep during the reading.

Katherine patted his hand, then looked over at me as if we'd known each other for some time, then down at Larry, on the sofa. "We won't worry if you do go to sleep."

"I'll just go on reading," I said, grateful for what Katherine had said, "if that's all right with you, Larry."

It was, of course. Larry settled in under his blanket. Katherine had to leave us. She had to dress to go to a memorial service for a colleague—he had died suddenly, in his sleep—to be held that afternoon in Tuskegee. I caught a glimpse of her kissing Larry on the forehead before she left the living room. Then, opening *The Hobbit*, I fastened my eyes on Chapter II, entitled "Roast Mutton." I didn't realize I had put "Pagoda" aside; in fact I didn't think of the story again.

I had the dwarves on their way with Bilbo Baggins, on the first day of their journey, when Larry's son Jason came into the living room. He was wearing a pair of baggy gray shorts, nothing else. Flaxen-haired, with a scraggly Viking's beard, a big-boy-not-yet-grown aspect to him, uneasy, overassertive, he didn't look like he had much going for him at age twenty-six. The model ship he was working on—*The U.S.S. Constitution*—was in a partial state of assembly on the coffee table by the sofa. Its spars were in place but not the rigging and sails.

I stopped reading and introduced myself without getting out of my chair. I complimented Jason on the model ship. Jason told me "Old Ironsides" came with prefabricated parts—all he had to do was assemble them. He didn't look like he wanted to stay long. He said he had to go to dialysis today. I asked him how many days he went, and he told me he had to go three days a week.

Then, abruptly, Jason went to his father, standing over him, beaming down at him. "You'd like me to be gone every day. That way, you could have the house to yourself."

Larry's smile was back; he was playing along with Jason. "There's too much house here for me to have by myself. But this sofa, that I do like to have for myself."

Jason kept the their little game going. "As far as I'm concerned, that sofa's got your name on it, Dad."

I was about to focus on the Happy Birthday balloons when Wiley the cat leapt onto the sofa. Jason grabbed Wiley; he had the cat bundled against his hairy chest. "No sir, Wiley; stay off the sofa. That's Dad's sofa, not yours, my man. You and me, we're moving on."

I watched Jason leave the living room, a firmly gripped Wiley peering over his shoulder. Jason would get dressed, get into his Trans-Am, make the five-mile drive to East Alabama Medical Center and go through having his blood drained out of a wrist fistula, purged of impurities in a dialysis machine. The clock was ticking; I was reading on. Katherine Beckwith came in, wearing heels and a tailored black suit. She kissed her husband tenderly. She told him she would be back by four. Then, unobtrusively, she left the living room.

I read the next chapter at a slow pace, doing patches of oafish troll dialogue, such as "poor little blighter let him go," with some semblance of Tolkienian gusto. I read on through Chapter II, how Bilbo and the dwarves escaped being devoured by the trolls and, shepherded by Gandalf, reached the land of the elves. Names I'd once known recovered their familiarity—Elrond the elf king, Gondalin, the Misty Mountain. It came back to me while I was reading—years ago, in the late sixties, I used to sit up reading *The Lord of the Rings* on those few nights I wasn't preparing for a class— smoking, nursing a watery drink, this was in 1968, when my children had their childhood ahead of them, when my marriage to Sandra, my second wife, looked like it might last. I would be sitting in another armchair, Sandra having gone to bed early (she taught in a private high school and had to be up at seven). I would be avidly following Tolkien's Hobbit hero, old Bilbo's grandson Frodo, in his stewardship of the ring of power, his long and bitter struggle with Sauron, the ruler of the dark kingdom of Mordor. What, I asked myself, had impelled me to read *The Lord of the Rings*; I mean read it through, all three books? There was the cold war, the bomb, the Soviet Union, the assassinations. It wasn't that hard to take a Manichean view in the late sixties, and then there was Tolkien's unlikely Middle Earth having some connection with the psychedelic business, Sergeant Pepper, marijuana, LSD. In the sixties, *The Lord of the Rings* had swept me along. As for *The Hobbit*, or so it seemed today, these trolls about to barbecue dwarves, these noble warrior elves, clever Gandalf—they didn't matter much to me now. Yet I read on, trying to inflect my voice, show some enthusiasm, while Larry Beckwith dozed, shifted his legs or fiddled with the tie to his bathrobe.

When I finished, closed up the book, Larry sat up on the sofa. "You read very well," he said, smiling. "Have you ever done any acting?"

"No, I haven't." Here was a chance to open up a little. "I was afraid to try out in high school. I didn't think I could memorize lines. You had to quote the Gettysburg Address to get into my high school drama club. That was all there was to it, but at the time it seemed too much for me."

Larry's smile softened; he seemed to understand that the little acting I'd done today had been for him. "Well, even though you're not an actor, I still think you read very well."

"Yes, I used to read aloud in class. I got a lot of practice teaching for thirty-four years."

"Well it certainly shows. I enjoyed it."

I was out of my chair, moving toward Larry, still sitting up, supporting himself with both hands on the arm of the sofa. When we shook hands, his right hand had to cross over his left to find my outstretched right hand. It was an awkwardly formal leave-taking we had on that day.

In my car, a block away down South Gay Street, I realized I'd left "Pagoda" behind. I decided not to go back and get it, for Larry might be asleep by this time. Later on, I called his home. Katherine Beckwith answered the telephone. She told me my story was in good hands. She would keep it for me, on the microwave.

LARRY BECKWITH DIED a week later, on the night before I had arranged to make my next visit. Katherine Beckwith telephoned Linda Merritt that morning, and, later on that day, Linda telephoned me. I said what I had to say, "I'm so sorry; I was going to see him today." I had taken the cordless telephone to the living room, looking out at the pecan tree in the front yard, its leaves edging into rhubarb red. The red flag was up on the mailbox. Linda's voice came back, close to her director of volunteers voice. Larry was an organ donor, so there would not be a funeral, nor a visitation at a funeral home. A memorial service would be held at Saint Andrew's Episcopal Church, in Tuskegee. Linda wasn't sure when, but when she found out she would let me know. I said something about Larry's condition; he'd seemed weak but not really that bad off. Linda told me she had heard that Larry didn't want to linger on through the last stages. He had told one of the nurses he didn't want his loved ones to have to go through seeing him get worse and worse. We talked on a little longer. Then I was holding the mute cordless, returning it to the receiver while the mailman delivered the mail and the pecan tree stirred in the October breeze.

What I wrote down then and there were my feelings about

Larry Beckwith's death. "As his passing sinks in, I'm inclined to think he's been spared the suffering and humiliation of the final stage. He didn't have to go through what Lonnie Simmons or Howard Carr did. And he did see his sister before he died. And a week ago he'd had a birthday party. He had just turned forty-eight. With me reading to him he heard only of the setting forth of Bilbo Baggins. He'd smiled over the two sides of Bilbo, the Took and the Baggins in him. He'll not hear of Bilbo's battle with the dragon, but maybe that's all right, for in my last reading Bilbo had reached the magic kingdom of those gentle warriors, the elves."

That was as far as I could go. Yes, I know, Disney World has a lock on magic kingdoms, but even Disney World goes beyond sheer escapism for a few minutes. Our shared magical landscape might have gone beyond solipsism, beyond J. Alfred Prufrock's "decisions and revisions which a moment can reverse." There are minutes that are not reversible; that much, I realized, had come home to me.

A little later Natalyn came in from her studio, and I told her what had happened. She was surprised and saddened by the news. We talked about calling Katherine Beckwith. I said I thought I should wait a day, but that evening I did call her. As soon as I heard her voice, calmly thanking me for my concern, I was glad I had done so. I said I was just getting to know Larry. "Yes," she replied, "I realized that you were becoming attached to him. And Larry appreciated the reading. There will be a memorial service," she informed me, "next Wednesday, on November 3, at Saint Andrew's Episcopal Church in Tuskegee. That's still our church," she went on to say, "even though we've been living in Auburn." I said I would certainly be there.

Larry Beckwith's sister, Jane Beckwith Mott, was standing at the left side of the chancel. Her voice trembled as she read out her tribute, tears in her eyes, looking up from the sheet of paper, looking out at the people in the church, deriving sustenance, the strength to go on, from them. At least two hundred people sat listening in the air-conditioned quiet. Many were members of the congregation, others were friends and colleagues from Tuskegee University. I don't want to paraphrase what Jane Mott said, or what her sister-in-law Louise Lippincott said. It has become a remembered tableau for me now, the spacious, light-flooded, Episcopal church, with its banner, the Cross of Saint Andrew, hanging down behind the altar, plush red seats on the whitened pews, the choir's red robes, the polished beams intersecting over the nave. The heartfelt tributes unfolded, revealing more and more of Larry's goodness. Yes, he was devoted, caring, self-sac- rificing—and now another woman, from Tuskegee Institute, an African-American colleague, spoke of Larry's willingness to take over her classes when she was ill, that and much else he had done. From the pulpit, on my right the priest delivered the eulogy. Toward the end, in a buoyant baritone he affirmed, "There were cheers in Heaven when Larry got there." Laughter rippled along the whitened pews, not much, just enough for a momentary lightening of mood.

A communion service followed the eulogy. I had the prayer book in my hands again, reading "The Apostles Creed," "The Prayers of the People"—it had been years since I'd taken communion. Today the family members took communion, but aside from two elderly white members of the congregation, no one else did.

After the service, the family members were assembled outside the open church doors. It took some time for everyone to file out, and while I waited, I noticed that the Indian woman in front of me had an elephant with a howdah patterned on her voluminous skirt. Four black teen girls, dreadlocks dangling, in fancy dresses, trooped dutifully after their parents. It seemed to take forever for both sides of the aisle to empty out, but at last I was getting close to Katherine Beckwith. She looked taller in her black suit—was it what she had worn the last time I'd seen her, before she went to that other memorial service? I approached her, and we lightly embraced.

"It was a lovely service."

"It was good of you to come," she said, then in the brief space of time that we lingered, "I still have your short story."

"I'll call you sometime and come get it."

I was moving on, along the line of family members. I shook hands with Jason, imposing in his blue suit, nodded and said something to the others. At last, I was moving away from the church, down stone steps to the parking lot.

I drove past the gates of Tuskegee Institute on the Montgomery Highway, taking state road 81 through the north side of Tuskegee. I stopped to go to the restroom at a Burger King, and on my way out to the parking lot, the Indian woman and her husband passed me going in, her howdahed skirt announcing a coincidence of sorts. I drove on out 81 to I-85 and, swinging off the entrance ramp onto the freeway, I found myself behind a speeding log truck, bunched logs slanting down, trailing its harsh red flag.

Several weeks went by before I saw Katherine Beckwith again. A week or so after the funeral, I left my number on the answering machine. I called again a week later, and again I heard her voice on the answering machine. After that I didn't call back for awhile, not until mid-November. This time Jason answered. He told me his mother was working. She must be in her office at the school, twenty miles away at Tuskegee Institute. Or was she in her own home, grading papers, preparing a lecture? Thanksgiving came and went. I called again. On an afternoon early in December I drove by the house. Jason's Trans-Am was parked in the front yard.

There was a white sedan parked in front of Larry's blue Mazda Miata—that must be Katherine Beckwith's car. But I didn't stop that afternoon; I had something else to do, errands to run, and then just dropping in, that would not be appropriate?

I came back a few days later, after dark, along about five PM. The white sedan was in the driveway, and a light was on in the kitchen. Another light burned in what must be a bedroom to the left of the front door. The blue-backed volumes of *The Journal of the American Chemical Society* were no longer stacked behind the box hedge, below the overhanging roof. I went to the kitchen door instead of the front door. It didn't seem that far from the front door, actually. Back when I was reading to Larry, the distance between the doors seemed greater.

Katherine Beckwith was facing the microwave; she had her back to me when I knocked. Turning, she saw me, a startled recognition flashing in her wary eyes. Then, smiling, she came to the door.

She was wearing black, or some fabric close to black, a blouse and slacks, her face pallid in the lemony fluorescent lights in the ceiling fixture. I said I'd come by to pick up the journal with my story in it, which I'd left behind the last time I had visited Larry. Katherine Beckwith picked the journal up off the microwave—yes, it was still where she'd put it on the day I last saw Larry Beckwith alive. She held it out to me, and I took it.

"Did you leave anything else?" she asked, knowing, I'm sure, that I hadn't.

"No that was all," was my answer.

As if she knew I wanted to apologize for not seeing her sooner, she said she wasn't at home that much at night, now that she was working again. I said I thought you might be out of town, and a shadow came over her face as sorrow took over. "Yes, I was out of town for awhile," she said to me. I didn't ask where, or when.

I sensed she didn't want me to talk any longer. But I couldn't just turn around and go. I remembered my friend, the Tuskegee Institute art professor, Ruth Morehouse, telling me she had gone to a concert given by the Auburn Chorale, in memory of Larry Beckwith. Ruth had missed Larry's memorial service; she was visiting her sister in California at the time. After a little while, I said I'd heard about the concert from Ruth Morehouse. Katherine told me it was very beautiful, that Larry would have liked it. Then she said, "There was a nice paragraph about Larry in the *O-A News.*"

We stood facing each other a little longer. "I hope you're doing all right," I said, finally.

"Yes I am," Katherine said, her voice enervated, played out. Yet she too seemed unwilling to say good-bye. "And you?"

I was doing all right, I said. Our eyes met, and I reached out and clasped her hand. We shook hands with excessive formality. Then, releasing my hand, as if she felt she should reassure me, she said, "And good luck to you."

"Good luck to you," I replied, no more than that.

Wishing each other good luck, that, I felt, had been serendipitous. It made it easier for us to say good-bye.

6

A Long-Stemmed Red Rose, Purchased at Kroger

S OMETHING WAS CHANGING at Eileen Foote's. I was spending more time with Cassie Binton than I had while while I was seeing Larry Beckwith. Late October and early November found me facing Eileen in the living room, leaning forward in the rocker in order to follow her drifting discourse, her trials and tribulations, her thoughts on raising children, the pernicious drug problem, her childhood and family memories, the minutes on the living room clock skittering by until it was time for us to see Cassie Binton again, to move from the living room's trophies and glass figurines to Cassie's bedroom, with its paint-peeling, flat blue, discouraging walls, the cluttered—no, overloaded—vanity, the aluminum rails of the confining hospital bed, the machine for draining urine and feces squatting silently between the beds.

I was still distanced from Cassie's condition, her addled sense of time, place, and circumstance. I could tell myself I was here for Eileen's benefit, as an auditor, a person she could talk to. Yes, I did see Cassie, and I talked to her some. I took her hand when I said hello and, taking my leave, I'd say, "See you next time." I'd already given her the Robert Forbes print, *December*. Now it was hanging on one of the bedroom walls. Its Kensington Gardens formality seemed unruffled by all the clutter. Even though it was hanging shakily from a Phillips-head screw, *December* had been able to accept its new home with equanimity.

Late in October, in a secondhand bookstore, I came across a poster with a still life subject. I named it, "Roses and Strawberries." On my next visit I presented it to Cassie.

"Do you like your picture?" I asked Cassie, "these are strawberries."

"Oh yes, well I declare," she said to me.

I duct-taped the poster beside Cassie's bed on the wall disfigured by the dangling strip of blue wallpaper. Cassie spit into the paper cup Eileen was quick to have ready for her. The poster had been taken down the next time I was there. Eileen prepared me for the poster's absence by saying she had to take it down, but her son James would tack it up somewhere else, which never happened. Just as well the thing went into the trash can. I came to associate *December* and "Roses and Strawberries" with the living room phase of my visiting, with Eileen's voice and manner, her stories, not with what I might term the later, bedroom phase.

We had warm days and chilly nights in the living room phase. Autumn was now in full swing, the golds of the elms and soft maples speckling the leaves that hadn't turned yet, the dogwoods flaring scarlet, dark red burnished oaks, the dried-out pods of the mimosas, a blue sky, sometimes a cloud-flannel sky. In the living room, Eileen shifted her feet in the green palmetto trimmed slippers, her eyes fixed on some distant focal point as she spun out another engaging story.

As a little girl, she had had to walk to school. No buses for us then, she told me. She walked to school. The school was four miles away if she went on the roads. To get to school on time, she had to cut through the woods and fields, cross over the creek a mile or so behind the house. She'd take her shoes and socks off and wade across. In the winter, the creek was iced over, so she'd have to crawl across on her hands and knees, with her book satchel strapped on her back, hoping and praying the ice wouldn't crack apart under her.

At age twelve she had been sent by her father to nurse a diabetic aunt. After her aunt died, her uncle—he had the sugar, too—wanted her to nurse him also. Eileen told her father, "I ain't goin'." Her father told her she didn't have to go. "I ain't goin'," Eileen reiterated indignantly, glaring at me as if she were faced with that choice again.

Another time she talked about her years in housekeeping at what was then known as Lee County Hospital. You cleaned up, dusted the Venetian blinds, mopped the floors and mopped them again when people tracked them up. She made $3.50 an hour with half an hour for lunch (she didn't offer this, I had to ask her what she made). Now that the hospital had more people in housekeeping , there was less work, and they didn't, she claimed, do a good job anymore. The housekeeping people today used only one bucket of water for mopping the floors.

When I asked her to tell me about her next job, at the laundry that at one time serviced the hospital (it has since been expanded, handling nursing homes as well the hospital, along with the new cancer center), she was happy to fill me in. She started her shift at 6 A.M. and got off at 3 P.M. She worked a machine for ironing and folding sheets. She would line up twenty wet sheets on the feeding tray, feed one in, and, moving to the other side of the machine, pick up the lengthwise folded sheet and flip it over—she demonstrated the movement with her hands—folding it end over end. If the sheet wasn't properly aligned before being fed into the machine, she would have to pull it out and fold it by hand. The folded sheets sliding out were still hot from the ironing. She showed me the palms of her hands; her skin was worn smooth, the palm lines standing out like tiny garter snakes. That's what the job had done to her hands. She pulled out a thousand hot sheets from that machine during an eight-hour shift, catchin' them, was what she called it. Looking out at me with a big grin, she said, "I still dream about catchin' all them sheets."

She went on to tell me that there were five women and five men working with her at the time. The men had it easier, for what they did was feed the dirty linen—sheets, contours, pillowcases, and towels—into the washers. The women had to help each other, and if a man was out on sick leave, help out with the washing too. She told me she helped her friend Mary fold the contours, pillowcases, and towels. These all had to be done by hand, and Mary could do it so well you'd never know the difference. But if Mary needed help, Eileen would pitch in. You worked until the job was done, helping others out when they got behind. She didn't mind work, and she liked the people she worked with. I asked her about her supervisors, and she told me once you figured out what their quirks were it wasn't hard to get along with them. They always treated her right, because they knew she didn't sit around on the job or take excess trips to the bathroom. It wasn't a bad place to work at all. And the meals the hospital would bring in for lunch, and for breakfast sometimes too, they gave you all you wanted to eat and drink.

She leaned back in the armchair, her face hazed in nostalgia, and said she'd like to go back there someday, see what the place was like now.

Eileen quit that job in 1992 to nurse her sick father. He had the sugar, too, and was going to dialysis three times a week. At that time, Cassie had been living in the house, with her sister Susie Mae. Cassie did the cooking, and had a garden, but after Susie Mae died, Cassie was never right in the head. "She wanted to be in the kitchen, do all the cooking herself, and she was turning the gas on all the time. We couldn't do nothing with her, and then she got the cancer and had to stay in her bed. In some ways, that made it easier for me."

Another time Eileen told me about tending to Cassie over the weekend (the bathing women, she made clear, came only during the week). She would wash Cassie while she was lying in bed, for Cassie would faint if you put her in a chair—the bathing women had tried to carry her in one—although sometimes she could lie propped up; that was due to the mucus in her throat. Eileen would get Cassie's nightgown off, change Cassie's diapers, and wash her parts thoroughly, then bathe her and dry her off and put on powder. Then she would slap baby oil all over her, to guard against bed sores. To change the bottom sheet, she would roll Cassie over on one side of the bed, pull the sheet out, roll Cassie to the other side, and ease the sheet out from beneath her fragile body. She'd put the clean bottom sheet on the same way. She claimed the Lord had come to her and shown her the way to do this.

Certainly, Eileen was a resourceful nurse. Cassie had a clean nightgown on every time I saw her. Whenever Cassie's throat was clogged with mucus, Eileen was there with the paper cup, and although she seemed a bit impatient with Cassie's maunderings—"No, it isn't Sunday, hon'; it's Tuesday," "no, you don't have to shell any peas today"—she never lost her temper or showed any lack of solicitude.

As I have indicated, Eileen's reminiscing, my listening interspersed with leading questions, characterized the living room phase of my visits. The bedroom phase must have started on the day I brought Cassie a dollar-ninety-nine long-stemmed red rose purchased at Kroger. I had arranged with Eileen to come on a Thursday, at the usual time, around 1 P.M. It was a warmish day in early November, two weeks after Larry Beckwith died. I had been keeping my visits with Eileen and Cassie detached from my visits with Larry Beckwith. At Eileen's, I didn't think of Larry stretched out on the sofa while I read to him from *The Hobbit*.

Pulling into the familiar front yard, the yellow fire hydrant behind me, I saw that the yard had been mowed. Eileen's car was not parked out in front; the house itself looked deserted. I had to tamp down a surge of resentment; Eileen had no business running off today, even though I was half an hour late getting here. I thought about coming back another time; then I saw a short black man, stout, with a grizzled beard, shuffling out of the shed behind the house. He wore a caved-in felt hat, its brim frayed at the edges. I moved on around the side of the house, the Kroger rose lowered, held casually. We met by the steps to the kitchen door. I introduced myself as Cassie's Hospice volunteer. He said he was a neighbor down the road, Homer Fisher. Eileen, he informed me, had gone to the doctor's. We shook hands, and I showed Homer the rose I was carrying, asking him if I could give it to Cassie.

"Yes, come on in," he said.

Homer let me in through the kitchen door. He escorted me to the bedroom, sitting down in a chair by the bedroom door. Cassie was wearing a light blue cotton nightgown. Her hair wasn't plaited today. I went up to her with the rose on display.

"It's for you," I said, taking her hand.

"Oh, that's nice," she said, beaming up at me.

Homer sat by the door without comment. I asked him if Eileen had a vase to put the rose in. He got up and said he would get something. He said he might have to trim the rose down before he could put it in water, so, reluctantly, I let him take it along. I was alone with Cassie for the first time. No change in the scaly blue wall, which drew my gaze hypnotically. I tried to say something Cassie could comprehend.

"Eileen tells me you have a big family, Cassie."

"Oh yes," she said, nothing more.

A pause, and then, "She tells me you had a garden once." Cassie didn't say anything to that.

I sat on the edge of Eileen's double bed, and some moments of silence went by. Cassie kept her hands folded over her stomach, breathing regularly, her crusted brown lips flapping open, the pink inner lip showing. I said something about the picture on the wall, *December*.

"Do you like your flowers?"

"Flowers. Oh yes," Cassie said, beaming up at me as she had when I showed her the rose. Presently, Homer Fisher came back with a lime-tinted plastic water glass half full of water, the rose poking out, short stemmed now. Homer didn't live here, but most certainly he'd taken over. Now he was handing the rose in its improvised vase on to me, motioning for me to set it on a bed tray toward the foot of Eileen's bed. That I did, without thinking twice about it.

I wrote a note to go with the rose, on a note pad I carried in my left hip pocket, for jotting down material I might use in a story. I knew my handwriting was bad. So I tore off a sheet of note paper, pressing it firmly against the pad, and slowly, meticulously, I printed out:

> For Cassie Binton and Eileen Foote
> from Charles Rose

Homer Fisher still sat in the chair by the door, beneath John Forbes's eighteenth-century *December* print, watching me set up the note on the bed table. He pushed the brim of his hat up a little. I folded the note paper vertically, propping half of it against the plastic water glass, Cassie's vase.

Still sitting on the edge of the bed, I tried to fill the silence somehow. I said to Cassie, "Thanksgiving will soon be here," but since Cassie had no notion of the time of year, this remark didn't register with her. I asked her if she missed her sister, Susie Mae. "I ain't seen her lately," Cassie replied. Homer Fisher listened to all this without comment. Eileen had some nice photographs of her children, I said, as much to Homer Fisher now as to Cassie. Perhaps Homer thought I was alluding to the photographs on the vanity, displaying two attractive preteen girls beaming out smiles for one and all, for he came back with "Yes, they're in the living room. These in here are Eileen's nieces."

It was becoming evident that Homer didn't want me to hang around much longer. Perhaps he wanted to be somewhere else himself, or perhaps my presence here put him off. Having a sixty-eight-year-old white man in his neighbor Eileen's bedroom, for Homer that was carrying goodwill too far. Still and all, I told myself, Cassie's rose had given her pleasure. Before I left, I'd show it to her again.

I held the rose out over her bed. Her eyes were open, she was attending.

"I hope you like your rose. And that you won't forget who gave it to you." Cassie gazed at the rose. Stretching her slack lips, she smiled up at me.

"I won't forget," she said. Then her eyelids were drooping again.

I put the rose back on the bed table, propped the note back up on the water glass. I said, "I'll see you next time, Cassie," but Cassie had already drifted off.

Homer escorted me to the living room. I tore another sheet from my note pad and printed out a note to Eileen.

2 PM
Dear Eileen,

Sorry I missed you and hope you're feeling better. I gave
Cassie a rose. I'll call you about visiting Wednesday or Thursday
of next week.

Charles Rose

Yes, I printed the note out meticulously while this poker-faced
black man stood in front of the flowered sofa, the crown of his hat
level with the glass figurines encased on the wall, the tabbies and
Santas, the feisty pups and gargantuan rooster, hands in pockets,
hat brim pulled down, eyes shadowed in dubious scrutiny. I put
the note on the table beside Eileen's armchair. I told Homer I'd
be on my way. Homer opened the front door and slipped the
catch to the storm door, then made room for me to push it open
and leave. He reached out and slowly pulled the storm door back
before easing the front door shut.

I WAS BACK AGAIN, sitting on the edge of Eileen's bed. Eileen sat
beside me, inches away. She was wearing a green sweater over a
sweatshirt, jeans, and canvas shoes (not the palm tree slippers).
The bed springs creaked from our combined weight. Cassie was
propped up on three pillows. Her left knee was raised, creating a
knobby bulge in the blanket.

Then Eileen went out to the kitchen to do something. I heard
her humming a hymn while I sat with Cassie. I told Cassie I was
going to bring her a Christmas present, and Cassie said, "that will
be nice" with this courtly intonation her voice had at times, her
ladylike good manners voice. She was quiet for awhile, her face in
repose, long-fingered, large gray fingernails, green nightgown, pale
green sheet, her bib, displaying Tweety the chipper cartoon bird,
tied in place. Clouds were visible through the slats of the Venetian
blinds, their slow drift. Astonishing, what Cassie said next—"I
miss my pies." She could have been saying that to Susie Mae.

Eileen was back. I made room for her on the double bed. Here we were, here was the little Tweety bird. Cassie was coughing again, Eileen was getting up, bending over her with the paper cup, Cassie spitting, more silence. Cassie wanted to know if they were picking cotton. Eileen looked at me, raising her eyebrows, we-know-better written all over her face for the span of a second or two. "Oh no, sug', it's past time for that." Cassie folded her hands, without comment.

I had to ask Eileen about cotton; was much raised around here? No, farther south was where cotton was raised. Now Eileen was talking about picking cotton when she was a girl. She didn't want any more of that. She'd have to drag a croker sack full of cotton and then load it on the cotton truck. Another reason she wouldn't want to pick cotton was the spray they used for boll weevils. She knew the poison in it had caused people to die. The fish were belly up in the creek. You could smell the spray seven miles off. The flowers, seemed like they wilted.

ON DECEMBER SIXTEENTH, I brought a poinsettia out for Cassie's Christmas present. I'd told her during my last visit, I'll bring you a Christmas present. It was an A&P poinsettia, not that large, not that red, not that rich in chlorophyll. I had also inked out a card, a Santa, six, not twelve, crudely sketched reindeer, legs every which way, antlers awry, Merry Christmas inscribed over Santa's cap.

On the sixteenth I took my gift out to Eileen's. It was sitting on the car seat beside me, this not quite pint-sized poinsettia. Out in front of the Lazy Bee was a sign garlanded with pine branches, a red ribbon trickling along the top. Merry Xmas, in big black letters. On fence posts and pine boles, no trespassing signs stood out in somber contrast to the Christmas spirit, at least ten of them between the turnoff and Eileen's house. Eileen's car was parked out in front. I got out and went to the passenger door, took the poinsettia out, cradling it carefully so the card, one corner wedged in poinsettia dirt, wouldn't come loose and tip over. When I knocked, I heard Eileen humming a lilting hymn on her way to answer the door. She was wearing a long-sleeved crew-necked grayish sweater with EAMC spread out in balloons, the balloon stems converging below her breasts on the rubric MEDICAL CENTER. I had no idea where the sweater came from.

Inside, in the living room, no Christmas tree, no decorations, not what you'd see in Auburn. Eileen held a paper cup with a straw, what looked like a milk shake—and a half-eaten hot dog smeared with mustard. She liked the poinsettia, appreciated my bringing it. We would take it on back to Cassie, she said. Cassie had had a bad night last night. Eileen had been up with Cassie until four in the morning. She had to use the machine to suck the mucus out, but today Cassie was doing better.

Eileen finished the last bite of hot dog, set the paper cup down beside her big armchair and led me back to the bedroom. Going in, I lifted the poinsettia up and held it out in front of me. Eileen stayed by the door. "Mister Rose is here to see you," she said.

Her face turned to the wall, Cassie was scratching her neck, with one hand, then another, her fingers digging down under the Tweety bib, her blunt gray nails imbedded in flesh. "Don't scratch your neck. Move your hands Cassie." Eileen went over to Cassie and moved her hands down to the blanket. She untied the strings of the Tweety bib, loosened it, and re-tied the bib. "That feel better?" Cassie kept her eyes on the wall.

I had to say something. "How you feelin' today?"

Cassie slowly turned toward me. "I'm feelin' all right."

Holding the poinsettia out over the bed, I lowered it over the furrows in the sheets, where her legs were, so Cassie could get a good look. "This is your Christmas present, Cassie."

"It's a poinsettia; isn't that pretty," Eileen chimed in.

"Isn't that nice," Cassie said, smiling.

"I told you I'd bring you a Christmas present. Remember? I told you that the last time I was here."

Her long fingers were touching, probing the foil an inch or so away from mine. I turned the foil so she could see the card. "And here is your card. It says 'Merry Christmas. To Cassie Binton from Charles Rose.'"

Through gaps in the poinsettia, we regarded each other in silence. Then, from Cassie, just as I was lifting the plant, moving it out from between us—"I'll take care of it," she said, looking straight at me now, so I'd know, I realized, that she meant what she said.

Not much left of the poinsettia, a few ragged, wilting leaves on two stems, bedded in foil-wrapped dirt. It was sitting on the crowded vanity, with the lotions and creams, the baby oil for Cassie's bedsores. We were in January of 1999. The sign outside the Lazy Bee read:

Have a good 1999. Wow! 2000 next.

Sitting with Cassie, I heard a conversation going on in the living room. "All these boys care about is sellin' drugs. They don't care about nothin'."

Eileen had a garrulous visitor in the living room. Whoever it was, a neighbor, a friend, was laying out her views on child raising, her abrasive, know-it-all voice carrying back to the bedroom. Eileen could hardly get a word in edgewise. "You can't play with kids. . . . I don't play peer with them. . . . They know enough not to talk on my phone."

Cassie had a blue towel draped over her neck and chest. She was lying quietly in her bed. I was sitting in the chair by the door, drawing an angel in the sky, with a Pilot V-Ball pen, fine point, on note paper from the pad I carried with me. Instead of reading to her, I was drawing for her, for I was convinced she couldn't follow a text.

I used to teach *Paradise Lost* in sophomore lit, back in the days when some exposure to Milton's epic was still required, and now Milton was cautioning me to keep this angel masculine, for all the angels in *Paradise Lost* were masculine. But since I wasn't sure that would suit Cassie, I fudged theologically, sketching out a quasi-androgynous angel, with flowing but not cascading hair, cartoon eyes with slightly curved lashes. My angel was wearing long robes ending in tiny feet. My he/she angel was clasping, much the way girls used to hold their clipboards and books in the days when I was in high school, a modest harp, a doughnut halo floating over her/his head.

When I finished, I tore the drawing out, making an even, if slightly serrated tear, got up, and started for the hospital bed to show Cassie the drawing. On the way, I bumped one of the metal bedposts at the foot of the bed. Cassie was quiet, but she noticed.

"Is your leg all right?" I heard her ask with concern.

"Yes, it's okay," I said, and moved on up to the head of the bed. "Looks like I bumped the bed."

"You all right?" she asked again, mumbling this time.

"I'm fine." I held the drawing out so she could see it. "I drew you an angel, Cassie."

From the living room came the abrasive voice: "Lots of people want to put their children before their marriage. I don't put my children before my husband."

Cassie moved her head on the pillows, her hands sliding off the blue towel. She smiled up at me. "Well, I declare."

I took one hand and slipped the drawing between her thumb

and forefinger. She scanned it, then turned it over so the blank side was visible to her now. "An angel. Isn't that nice," she said.

I waited a little while before I took Cassie's hand and turned the sheet of paper around so she could see the drawing. "Look, he has a halo. And a long robe and wings."

"Yes, don't he now."

So the angel turned out to be masculine after all. Not long before Eileen came back, Cassie did something unpredictable. She rolled the drawing up lengthwise into a cylinder, and placing the fingers of each hand over it, she held it possessively, her concave, crudely drawn angel inside her scroll, curving into the curve of the sky. I caught a glimpse of the doughnut halo.

THE POINSETTIA WAS STILL on Eileen's vanity when I made my visit on January fourteenth. A few ragged leaves were left, spots of vermilion peeping out from the colossal clutter. When I arrived, Eileen told me Cassie had had diarrhea for four days. Eileen was feeding her Gatorade and warm milk, out of a syringe, into Cassie's PEG tube, along with the usual painkiller. Cassie was visibly weaker, and from what I saw, she must have been having cramps in her belly. Her lips were pulled in, twisted like rope, her neck wrenched to one side, her eyes squinched up. Pretty soon the pain eased up, and I took her hand and told her I was sorry she was feeling bad.

I was only there for a few minutes. Before I left I said to her, "I'll see you later, Cassie."

She replied in her old-fashioned, mannerly way. "All right. Do so then."

A nurse came by not long after Eileen and I left the bedroom. The nurse had two new Hospice volunteers with her. A black woman with a stethoscope dangling out of one ear, she looked vaguely familiar. She didn't know my name, but she knew who I was, for she'd seen me at one of the training sessions. She was the nurse, I remembered her now, replete in savvy and good will, who had talked about alleviating pain. The volunteers, a pallid young man wearing glasses and a gawky blond girl with acne, shuffled uneasily in the bedroom. The nurse told Eileen to give Cassie Immodium, and to call her if Cassie was not better by tomorrow.

Eileen talked a lot that day. "I do love talking to you," she told me, and she meant it. She'd had a bad four nights, and needed to talk. At one point, her Uncle Tim shuffled in from the kitchen. He went on back to the bedroom, and a few minutes later passed us on his way out, without a word, without even looking our way. Eileen told me she didn't know what to do with Tim. Not long ago, Tim had gone to sleep in his trailer out back, with a pan of grits burning on the stove. Smoke was pouring out of the trailer; he could have suffocated, she was telling me.

She went into a long rambling account of her trip to Seattle for James's bone marrow transplant, repeating things she'd told me before. A white woman out there had asked her to pray for her cancer-stricken husband's tender body, how the Lord had showed her the way. And later on when James's gut was hurting and he was throwing up a lot, the Lord told her to press his belly, and she realized James was constipated. She took him to the hospital for an X-ray, and it turned out James was constipated. A nurse told her she should be a doctor, and she told the nurse she didn't have to have a doctor; she had a man she could talk to, and that man was Jesus. The VA had paid for everything, including airfare and housing. Because James had gotten cancer while he was in the Navy, the Navy made sure he got treatment.

I learned more about Eileen's daughter, Julia. Julia had worked her way through college in Atlanta, without help from Eileen, and, now that she had this good job with the telephone company, she was thinking of going to graduate school. She called Eileen twice a week, which was more than my daughters did, I said, although they called me more than I called them. I realized another living room phase was underway now, yet this time I was getting the feeling we talked just to be talking sometimes, with awkward pauses, gropings for something to say.

"NO SUGAR DOLL, we don't have no pecans anymore."

"I want Tim to bring me pee-cans."

"Quit talkin' like that, baby. Tim don't grow no pecans."

"Ohhh—kegh. You ask him to bring me some peanuts."

"Honey, you know we ain't grown peanuts since granddaddy was alive."

Coming in, I saw the poinsettia was where it had been. Cassie's head seemed too big for her body that day. I bent over the bed, took Cassie's hand. "I'm glad to hear you're feeling better today." She was better, in fact livelier than I'd seen her before. "I feel pretty good," she said back to me, and as I stepped back, she looked right at me and said, "How's your mother?" I felt confusion and sadness take hold of me, for my mother had died in 1986.

"My mother passed away thirteen years ago." Cassie's face fell, and Eileen let out a long sigh. "I have a brother and a cousin left in my immediate family."

Eileen said her family had dwindled, too. Cassie was still looking at me; she must have been following what we said, so I said I missed my mother. I said she lived a long time, but then I couldn't say more.

Pretty soon Eileen said Cassie needed to rest. Eileen had soup on in the kitchen. I thought of leaving, but since Eileen hadn't asked me to, I sat in the living room for awhile. Eileen and I made increasingly pointless small talk for about fifteen minutes, with raised voices, from kitchen to living room and living room to kitchen. I heard grease popping in a skillet, and then Eileen's snick-snick-snick chopping knife stopped, and I heard another voice in the kitchen.

"Just the Hospice person visiting," I heard Eileen say—to none other than Homer Fisher. Yes, he was standing in the kitchen door. Our eyes met in recognition; then I found my way to the door.

HALF AWAKE, WINDY OUTSIDE, another day. Above the paneled half-curtains billowing in the half-open bedroom window, I watched leaves fluttering beyond the dirt-streaked glass, white speckled gray branches, a wedge of gray sky above the aluminum siding of the house next door. Natalyn was in her studio; she had started painting again after weeks of frustrating inactivity.

I thought of Cassie Binton in a bed miles away from where I was now. She had asked me how my mother was? These same Wal-Mart or Big Lots paneled curtains had been in Lonnie Johnson's house. Now they were floating out, being pulled in against the frame.

Early in January I did a quick pencil sketch of Eileen's house, sitting in the front seat of my car, noting the brick foundation, plum-colored for me, the washed-out gray of the shingling, the shoe-polish tan of the front door with its three window slits in echelon, the concrete mushroom-like picnic table out back on one side of the wash house shed. During the week, I put in a flat blue sky, yellow sun-flecked ballooning cumulus clouds penetrated by sun-slashed olive drab jack pines, the Y-split, clay buffed drive, one arm of which led to the washhouse, the other to Uncle Tim's trailer (Tim dozing, hot grits smoking on the burner, perchance?) meticulously limned yet subdued rows of bricks—in living color, wielding my trusty watercolor pens devoid of nuance, hard to go wrong with, broad strokes here, crosshatching there, rubbed smudges evoking the front yard's matted grass. It wasn't long before the Foote house took shape, not bad for an erstwhile high school art student, strictly manqué, who had gone on to doodle cartoon figures.

My cartoon figures had gone back to childhood, persisted on up to the present. I drew, and sometimes colored, figures of horses, women (voluptuous), and men (heroic), in college classes, in the flyleaves of books during long bus rides, in the army nursing a 3.2 percent beer at the NCO club, through long-winded seminar reports while I was in graduate school. I drew men in uniform, Napoleonic grenadiers, cuirassiers, hussars, Roman legionnaires, French Foreign Legionnaires, Federals in blue, Confederates in gray, I even sent cartoons off to *The New Yorker* and *The Saturday Evening Post*. Nothing came of that but rejection slips. The sketching, the doodling increased once I got back to writing again in the early nineties. Most of my recent short stories had developed out of crude sketches, hen-tracked with nearly indecipherable commentary.

I hadn't done any landscapes, no sun-splashed olive drab pines, not for me then, for I failed at landscapes before, at my desk in this high school art class, where landscapes in colored pencil were obligatory, and, mind you, with the shadows right, the perspective, the pen or pencil strokes on even keel, the watercolors mixed right in the paint pan.

Looking over my drawing of the Foote house, I thought of my high school art teacher, Bernice McKinley, a lonely spinster who lived in the Courtland Hotel in Kokomo, on North Main Street across from the Indiana theater. On a summer evening, one might see her out on the balcony, in a rocker, it must have been a rocker, alone up there over the porticoed entrance, gazing out at the fading traffic, at the movie marquee in the fading light. She went to Brown County in the fall to sketch the turning leaves, took the weekend off and drove to Bloomington. She was perky in the classroom, her eyes crinkling when something tickled her.

She told me my work had some originality, but, unfortunately, I hadn't learned how to put the shadows in. She was right, I hadn't learned how to put them in. So I kept on doing cartoons, no need for shadows anymore. Until now. I had to try and put them in to achieve a measure of verisimilitude. Looking over the drawing one last time, I realized the shadows still weren't there.

A SUNNY DAY, late in January, sunlight filtering through the Venetian blinds. The poinsettia wasn't on the vanity anymore; it was sitting on the bed table. Cassie had had a bad night last night, but today she was feeling better. She was lying quietly in the bed, in a pink nightgown, her head propped up on two dark blue fluffy pillows. The tip of one of her braids was curled up and around so it grazed her forehead below the hairline. She gave me a smile when I came in, and I took her hand, as usual. Eileen sat on her bed, by the window.

"You look well today," Cassie offered, right away.

"Well, thank you. You're looking well too."

We talked some, and after a little while Cassie confused me with someone named Fred, who, Eileen had to tell her, was long gone, not for Cassie to worry about. It was time to present my picture. When I showed the picture to Eileen in the living room, she seemed pleased. She said she liked it and wanted to frame it, and I said I'd have it framed myself and bring it back to her next week.

I held the picture out so Cassie could see it and said, "It's a picture of your house, Cassie."

She took the picture and turned it over, scrutinizing her house topsy turvy. I had to turn it back right side up again for her. And say emphatically, raising my voice some:

"It's your house. It's where you grew up, Cassie."

Cassie's face wrinkled up in delight. "Oh that's my house, My house!"

Enthusiastic myself, I pointed out the bedroom on one side of the house, the window with aquamarine shutters. "Look, there's your bedroom."

"Well, I declare."

After I propped the picture up, against the lamp on the vanity, I became aware of something oddly resilient about the poinsettia I'd given up on last week. It looked healthy this week, sitting amid the vanity's clutter, sunlight beaming in on it. Eileen came out with some poinsettia news. "That plant looks like it's doing fine. One of the green leaves is already turning red."

Two stems, a few vermilion leaves scattered above on each, the leaves below olive green, one of which, yes, one of which showed, along one tapered side, a stippled blush of nascent vermilion. What had I known about a poinsettia? It was just another part of Christmas for me.

I asked Eileen how long it would take for the leaves to turn red. "About seven days, maybe eight," she replied.

"That poinsettia," I said, "is really doing well. Last week I thought it was on its last legs, and now look at it, it's doing fine. Isn't that remarkable?"

"Sometimes." Eileen said, "a plant will wither away, and sometimes it will keep on doing fine."

"I guess sitting where it is now," I had to say, "the sunlight could get to it."

"I've been keeping it watered," she said firmly. That was the end of our poinsettia talk. We turned our attention to Cassie again.

7

"I've Been Privileged To Be With Her"

ISS LUDEE AND MISS EARLEAN, they couldn't both have wanted that carpet of mine." Lalia Boone raised her eyebrows. "Here's what I wanted to tell Miss Earlean. 'When I offered to give you my carpet you said you'd make do with the carpet you have, but now that I gave it to Miss Ludee you want it back.'"

Linda Merritt was sitting beside me in the Hospice building conference room. Across the long, glassed-over conference table, mirror images of Lalia Boone and three other women, Agnes Terrell, a middle-aged, genteel, soft-spoken woman; Jean Jackson, an earnest, reserved, young matron who did much charitable work in the community; and the coed who had come in late, Nancy Whitfield, shy, self-effacing. Viewed through the conference table glass, the heads and torsoes of my colleagues were upside down like my own. What they would have seen on my side of the table, if they had been looking, was the head and torso of an older man, unkempt, unruly hair streaked with gray. Or, sitting beside me, a reversed Linda Merritt, her tightly curled light brown hair, ovaled face, rounded shoulders, and modest bosom. Upside-down mirror images of ordinary people at a 5 P.M. meeting on Monday, plates of cookies, diet drink cans leaving rings on the glass. In the unremitting fluorescent lights, I was reminded of a line from a poem by Theodore Roethke, yes, it was "Dolor": "I have known the inexorable sadness of pencils, neat in their boxes, dolor of pad and paper weight. . . ." Yet something was livening up the institutional atmosphere—telling stories about our Hospice experiences.

Lalia Boone went on with her story. I thought of what she'd told her husband, which she had reiterated for us a few minutes ago—"I told my husband I just couldn't live with that carpet of ours one day longer," meaning I want a new carpet soon, and the old one I want in the pickup truck so I can take it twenty-five miles up the road to LaFayette and give it to my Hospice patient, Miss Earlean Lacy. In that beginning phase of her story, I had envisioned Lalia driving the pickup—she wouldn't have asked her husband to do that—wearing khaki pants, denim shirttail hanging out, Dolly Parton on the tape player, the only white woman driving a pickup truck—that she'd made clear—in the southeast corner of LaFayette. Miss Ludee lived behind Jeffers Funeral Home, and Miss Earlean lived across the street, so, as Miss Ludee saw it, when the time came for the Lord to take her, her mortal remains wouldn't have far to go. All the undertaker had to do was park the hearse in front of her place.

Transporting the carpet from Miss Ludee's house to Miss Earlean's house wouldn't be difficult either. If Miss Earlean had to have the carpet in her house, all she had to do was ask her brother, John Harmon, to go get it.

"I knew when I talked to Miss Ludee that John Harmon would worm that carpet out of her. All Miss Earlean had to do was ask him because, as Miss Ludee says, Miss Earlean would always be his favorite sister. But I had to ask myself—what could I say to Miss Earlean to make her not want Miss Ludee's carpet just because it belongs to Miss Ludee now? Because originally I gave the carpet to Miss Earlean. What was I going to do?"

After the meeting, I went next door to Touchdown's to empty my bladder. I might have a beer, I told myself, if I saw anyone I knew. I'd been to Touchdown's one time last summer, after playing tennis on Wednesday night—in a men's doubles league, most members of which were between twenty-five and forty-five. My partner at that time, Bobby White, an education professor looking forward to retirement, was fifty-eight, and like myself, an old married man.

One night after we won one set and lost one instead of, as usual, losing two, Bobby persuaded me to tag along with some of the younger players who were adjourning to Touchdown's. We split a pitcher of beer, and talked about what it was like to play doubles at our age, but it wasn't long before we ran out of things to say—how much can you talk about university politics or Auburn football? We watched the Braves play the Padres, finished the pitcher, and went our separate ways.

Now five months later, I pushed open the swinging doors, which featured miniature baseball bats for handles, pausing to take in the clamor and smoke, the waitresses, the basketball game on the television sets. I spotted Bill Wanamaker drinking a beer at the bar. A big man with sloping shoulders, gray hair, salt and pepper beard, the cuffs of his striped shirt rolled back, he had the slouched stolidity of a man who is doing his drinking alone. As it happened, Bill was pleased to see me. I said I'd been to the Monday night meeting, and he said, "Well, you probably need a beer. All those cookies get to you after awhile."

I worked on a Michelob Light while Bill filled me in on his new position. He hadn't been public relations director for Hospice for awhile. At present, he was program director at a fledgling Auburn radio station, WENL. He had to be at work by 4 A.M., that was six days a week, rain or shine, from 4 A.M. to 4 P.M. He didn't like the hours, but he thought he had an opportunity to do some things. He had a half-hour spot in mind for creative people to talk about their work, "writers, for instance, like yourself," the director of the new community theater, the president of the Auburn Arts Association, some area painters and sculptors, and Dave Fassbinder, a chemistry professor who plays modern jazz piano. Dave had started a group recently, young guys who liked modern jazz and wanted to play together. I'd heard them knock out "All the Things You Are" at a rapid clip with no clinkers, and go on to do some good things. This at their first gig in a downtown bar, but since the audience, unfortunately, was minuscule, it had turned out to be their last.

Not much on the radio anymore, I was telling Bill. At one time the venerable Auburn station, WAUD, which went back to before I came to Auburn, was both popular and lively, thanks to the manager, the knowledgeable (about almost everything: old movies, growing up in Alabama, jazz, and swing) and irrepressible Bob Sanders. Bob played pop songs and swing from the '30s and '40s; he did fifteen minutes of classifieds followed by lost-and-found pets from seven-thirty to eight, salting both endeavors with witty asides. Since Bob retired and the station had changed ownership, WAUD had become almost exclusively a sports station. And the Opelika station, WJHO, largely featured gospel music and talk radio savants.

Bill told me what he was programing at WENL—sports call-ins, a lost-and-found spot, deejayed golden oldies from the sixties, some vintage country, along with Paul Harvey and Sally Jesse Raphael. But no Rush Limbaugh; no way, Bill said vehemently, let that Opelika Jesus station carry Rush Limbaugh.

I brought up my friend Madison Jones, author of ten novels about the South and recipient of quite a few literary awards, including, most recently, the T. S. Eliot Award. If you're looking for a writer, you might try Madison first, I suggested, but, I added modestly, once you get this project underway, I would be happy to be a part of it.

By this time I'd gone through one Michelob Light. I might be liking the fit of the bar stool, but one more and I'd be on my way. Halfway through that second Michelob, I let it slip out: I thought I might have the makings of a book—about the people I'd been with, the impressions I'd carried away with me, for instance Howard Carr's squawky beseeching voice when he tried to lift himself off the bed, Larry Beckwith dozing on the sofa, Cassie Binton exclaiming "Well I declare." I'd started writing things down, taking notes, sketching out images in a sketch book I kept in the car. I'd started doing this after Lonnie Simmons died. But now that I was involved in the writing itself, I was beginning to have second thoughts.

Bill fastened an appraising stare on me, then a loose smile fluffed out a fringe of his beard. "Why second thoughts? What you're doing sounds great to me. I mean what you're writing about, this stuff is real, you should be getting it down."

"I know. I keep telling myself that. But the thing is, in order to write about all this, I have to back off, I have to detach myself. I may even *want* to detach myself."

"That might happen to you anyway." Bill's elbows were on the bar, his left fist folded into his cupped right hand. "And another thing, the people you're with, you're seeing them the way they are. That you have to do to write about them." He cracked his knuckles, then let his right hand relax without disturbing his fisted left hand.

Howard Carr, his limp hands, Lonnie Simmons gasping for breath. "You're right and you're wrong about that, Bill. It's true, I'm seeing what's there, while I'm seeing it, some of that gets down on paper. But in the process of getting it down—what I feel, absorb, yes with intensity sometimes, has to be distanced if it's ever going to be gotten down at all." On the television screen, a one-handed push shot ripped the net, three points, briefly noted by both of us viewers.

Bill maneuvered his legs and body into another sitting position. "So that's something you'll have to live with. Seems to me you've been able to do that or you wouldn't be telling me about it now." His left fist was back in his cupped right hand, his elbows pushed in against his ribs. He gazed at me steadily, making sure I would heed what he had to say. "Look here, when we were with Lonnie Simmons, you remember, I said something to him, like who you were, that you'd be seeing him. We have no way of knowing what went on in his brain. But I do know this—something went on. I know I felt something present in that room, and I'm pretty sure you did too. What I'm trying to say is this. Lonnie, any one of these people we think of as terminal, as out of it, they're aware of something we aren't, there's something they could tell us if they had some way to get it out." Bill kept his gaze on me; I was listening. "They can't tell us, so we have to tune into it. But I will say this: Lonnie Simmons knew you were there, Dr. Rose."

I thought of Howard Carr pointing his finger at me—*leave-Iwantyou to leave!* And Larry Beckwith—*did you do any acting?* And Cassie Binton—*how's your mother?*

"All right, something was going on. I'm with you on that." That was as much as I could say.

Bill cracked his knuckles and drank the rest of his beer. "You don't have to say any more, Dr. Rose." Bill had an evening ahead of him to get through, a basketball game he wouldn't mind watching. His eyes were roaming off to flag the bartender, and I glanced at the basketball game on the television screen, and drank up and said I had to move on.

Bill's eyes took on his usual jocular glint; he had a loose smile, lips curling into his beard. "Just keep on paying attention; that way you'll have to go on writing," he said. "When you can't go on, that's when you'll have to stop."

But that wasn't yet, I said to myself, outside Touchdown's, on my way back next door to locate my car. The lights were off in the parking lot now that the Hospice people had gone home.

ANOTHER MONDAY NIGHT MEETING. Outside the conference room a vacuum cleaner whined. Lalia Boone was not here for this meeting. I sat at one end of the table; Jean Jackson sat at the other end. To her right, her image reflected like Jean's in the tabletop's glass, Agnes Terrell showed her usual composure. Beside me, to my right, the shy coed, Nancy Whitfield.

A recent volunteer, Lori Lassiter, sat between Agnes and Nancy. I'd met her in Linda Merritt's office. Another coed—in a slouchy T-shirt that made her neck look long, pale blond hair in a raggedy page boy—she'd been out with Linda to see Eileen Foote last week. The idea was she would sit with Cassie Binton so Eileen could get one or two hours rest. Eileen would rather have a woman there, Linda had explained with some embarrassment, while she was resting. Lori would spend some time with her on Wednesday, and I'd continue to see Eileen on Thursday.

Someone I hadn't met sat on my left, a stocky middle-aged man with a shiny bald spot. He was brimming over with vigorous goodwill. Introducing himself as Rob Waters, he asked me right off what I did. I said I was a former college professor. Oh yes, and what field were you in? I said I was in modern literature. And what do you think of Thomas Hardy's poetry? He liked it better than Hardy's other work, he said. I said I liked Thomas Hardy's poetry (my wife's favorite poem was Hardy's "Neutral Tones"). I didn't tell him Thomas Hardy had lost his faith after he read Charles Darwin on evolution, for Rob Waters was clearly bent on getting something back, if not belief in God, at least a belief in the good. That alone was enough to make me like him.

No plates of cookies tonight, or Diet Coke cans, but Linda Merritt did have a handout for us concerning the topic for tonight, intimacy with the patient. The handout contained a poem, entitled "Companioning." Linda started the meeting by reading it through, not an easy task for someone with an MFA in poetry, but she managed it, made it sound as good as it ever would sound. The last verse went like this:

> Companioning is about
> Listening with the heart, it is not
> About analyzing with the head.

The other stanzas were in much the same vein, hortatory, loaded with cliches like "sacred silence," "loving presence." Each stanza began with the word companioning, which, I was telling myself, was not a word at all. Later that night, I looked it up in a dictionary. *Companioning* was a present participle. The derivation of companion, to my crestfallen surprise, was, in Vulgar Latin, "one who breaks bread with another." But at the meeting I was on edge, verging on irritable, the vacuum cleaner grinding and whining outside, fluorescent light-motes sifting down on us, mirror images on the glass top to my right, yet, curiously, not on my left. Behind Jean Jackson a narrow window threw its image down on the tabletop, broken up by a band of glowing fluorescence like a guillotine blade about to crash down.

> Companioning is about being
> Still; it is not about frantic
> Movement forward.

The door opened and whoever was doing the vacuuming said

he'd be finished in a little while. It wasn't long before the vacuuming stopped. That made it easier for me to listen.

Apropos companioning, Agnes Terrell began talking about touching, just sitting there with her patient and friend, holding her hand, keeping silent. Surely Agnes hadn't been wearing what she had on tonight, a madras blouse, a tailored ankle-length skirt, a light glaze of powder, touch of rouge on her face, but for a little while she communicated how she'd felt with another woman's hand in her own. I remembered Howard Carr's limp hand in mine, my hand on the back of his neck supporting him while he had tried to raise himself out of his bed.

To my left, Rob Waters's voice barging in, hale and hearty Rob Waters interjecting, "What you're saying, Agnes, about touching, that's easier for a woman. It's tough for a guy to do that. We'd a lot rather do the handshaking thing." Rob was on his feet, putting on a demonstration, pumping his outstretched right hand. "Like we're really pushing each other away, at least keeping this wall between us." Rob was elaborating on other ways men could touch, the bear hug, the arm grip, but not many men would be holding hands. He had risen in place to make his point, his left hand clasping his right so we could visualize what meaningful touching was between one man, the caring volunteer, and one less-than-a-man, the male patient. He turned his head to put me into it. "That's not easy, believe me," fingers interlocked, not exactly wringing his hands, nor could you say he was praying either. "What you're describing, Agnes, just letting yourself go through touching, I find that very difficult. I find I have to focus very hard on being open with another guy. I'm not making that much progress, but I want you to know I'm trying." The women gazed at him commiseratively.

Rob was sinking down into his chair. I marked the fluorescence gilding his tonsured pate, and in fact, had he been cassocked and sandaled, he might have passed for a monk or a friar, hairy-chested, chock full of fellowship. But I soon realized it was meanspirited to be ridiculing Rob, for he was really serious about what he believed.

"I'm getting there," Rob said, "but it ain't easy." He looked over at me for confirmation.

"That's right," I said, with a squint-eyed smile, "I've got a long way to go myself."

The women still had their eyes on Rob, but I could tell they expected me to be next. I said sometimes touching just came about, and when it did, well it did, that's all. Men touching, I didn't go into it much. I didn't bring up holding Howard Carr's hand, for neither one of us would have wanted that if Howard had been in better shape.

The talk about touching soon played out.

Since Linda Merritt seemed unsure of what to say next, Agnes Terrell tried to keep the ball rolling. Somehow she got on hospitals. If a patient has to go back for treatment, how important it was for a volunteer to dispel the fear many people have of seeing their loved ones in a hospital. Hospitals could be frightening. And there was the dread of never coming out.

After Agnes finished, I felt apathy settle on me. And yet, a little later, something remarkable took place. It began when Linda Merritt asked the shy coed, Nancy Whitfield, to fill us in on what she had been doing as a volunteer. "You might want to talk about Katie Munson," Linda went on, glancing at Agnes. Agnes Terrell leaned across Lori Lassiter, giving Nancy a smile of encouragement. "I'd love to hear what you've been doing, Nancy."

For a little while Nancy seemed flustered. Gripping a key chain for her car keys in her left hand, she pinched colored tabs on the chain with her thumb. Her voice started out tentative. "Miss Katie Munson, she's ninety-one years old." Obviously nervous, her eyelids lowered, Nancy spoke in disconnected phrases at first. "I don't go out to see her that much. Sometimes I talk to her on the telephone." A long pause, but we were listening. Something now about the last time Nancy was there, what Mister Ben, Miss Katie's son, said about the peach tree blooming in the back yard. "It was blooming too early, was what Mister Ben said. A peach tree shouldn't be blooming in February." As an image of Katie Munson began to take shape for us, Nancy gained more confidence. Her fingers might be squeezing her key chain, but her eyes had a shine in them.

"Miss Katie places everything that happened to her as—before she lost her legs and after she lost her legs." Nancy told us Miss Katie had been in a wheelchair for years, diabetes had ruined her legs but that really didn't bother her. "She's always asking me what I'm doing. I'll call her up to ask how she's doing but she won't let me talk about her long. She wants to know what I'm doing." Another pause, then her voice picking up, "Miss Katie is ninety-one years old. She told me her mama remembered when the slaves were freed. Her grandmother was a slave woman; yes, I realize this may surprise you, her grandfather, he was the master. I mean I've read about this in history books, but when I heard Miss Katie telling me this, for the first time it became real for me." Nancy's fingers relaxed on the key chain, the jammed together colored tabs.

Another pause, and then—"I've been privileged to be with her."

Privileged, that was the word Nancy used. Now she waited for comments from us. Rob Waters spoke of Katie Munson's long life, moving "from the Wright Brothers to the space shuttle." Linda Merritt said that this woman was living during the stock market crash in 1929. She had so much to say, such a story to tell. Nancy said she wouldn't forget her, not after what they had shared. Agnes Terrell took a deep breath and said, "as long as someone remembers you, you are immortal." Turning to Nancy Whitfield, I tried to convey my own appreciation, with a smile, a few inadequate words. I don't think she realized how much I appreciated what she was saying.

Jean Jackson told us how important her memories of her grandmother had been for her. Jean's grandmother had died on Jean's birthday. She could remember her grandmother when she was a child. After her grandmother died, every year on her birthday, her mother and father took Jean and her brother to the grave site. They'd lay flowers on the grave and say a prayer. "It wasn't gloomy or morbid," Jean said, "not what you might think it was." It made her birthday mean more to her, because her grandmother was a part of it.

Nancy Whitfield didn't say much more. She did say Miss Katie never felt sorry for herself, even though she was ill and had lost her legs. "Of course if Mister Ben or anyone in her family asked her to do something she didn't want to do, she'd say 'don't you forget I ain't got no legs.'"

It wasn't long before Linda Merritt was thanking us for coming. I think we all felt we were a little less far apart at the end of the meeting than we were at the beginning. This time I didn't stop off at Touchdown's. Standing in the parking lot, I decided not to. I took a last look at the green neon tubes on the A-frame structure, taking note of the special for tonight:

CHICKEN WINGS
.25 A WING

8

From March to December

CASSIE BINTON DIED on October 20, 1999. The last time I was with her, in late September, she was lying quietly in her hospital bed, her hands folded over her nightgown. She wasn't kneading her gums. Before we went back to see her, Eileen told me Cassie wasn't doing well. She was sleeping a lot, she wasn't saying much. And her right arm had stiffened. When Eileen turned Cassie to change the sheets, Cassie's body would also stiffen. How long she would live, that, Eileen told me, was for the Lord to decide.

The first thing Eileen did when we got to the bedroom was drain mucus out of Cassie's esophagus. Eileen forced Cassie's head back and inserted a plastic tube into Cassie's mouth. The squat machine on the floor hummed, slurped a tobacco brown liquid into a Tupperware-like container.

I sat on the edge of Eileen's double bed, my eyes on the gash in the sickly blue wallpaper. You'd think Eileen would have pulled this dangling excrescence off the wall. I held a red camellia, which I had picked from the camellia bush in our back yard, in a green glazed vase. I looked down at the camellia, then out through the bedroom window at the inaccessible blue wash of sky beyond the stand of pines across the road. Finally, Eileen worked the tube out of Cassie's mouth. Cassie's lower lip sagged, her eyes showed relief.

Eileen propped Cassie's head on the pillows. Cassie's legs ridged the thin cotton blanket, one tight braid curled over her right ear. Eileen looked at me, holding the vase, then back at Cassie. "Mister Rose brought you a pretty flower, sug."

I got up from the bed, leaned over the railing. I held the vase out close to Cassie's hands. Her fingers, groping to find the vase, made a tentative contact with mine. I said something—I brought you a camellia—inadequate, not enough. Cassie's fingers closed on the vase. We both held it, fingertips touching, our eyes on the red camellia.

"Thank you," Cassie whispered. Those were the last words I heard her utter.

Between March and October of 1999, I visited Cassie and Eileen eleven times, fairly regularly until June 21. I have noted the dates: March 11, March 18, April 1, April 15, April 27, May 20, June 3, June 21. I didn't see Cassie again until August 31. I saw her on September 16, and after a one week interval I made my last visit on September 23. Prior to March 11, I was visiting Cassie every other week, sometimes every week. I have a reason for my subsequent neglect, one worth going into.

Toward the end of March, Natalyn and I put up earnest money on a house, a much larger house than we lived in, on a bigger lot, with many more trees, deciduous and evergreen. Beyond glass doors and clerestory windows, a woodsy, pie-shaped back yard would distance us from our neighbors. This house had built in bookshelves, two large bathrooms with glass shower doors, a fireplace, a long screened-in porch, a storeroom, a laundry room. For fifteen years we had gotten along pretty well in the seven-room, one-bathroom house we bought in 1985, seven small rooms and an exceedingly narrow bathroom, a small screened-in back porch. The house came with a sizeable detached double garage, which we had converted into a studio for Natalyn. By the time I became involved in Hospice, it was evident the house was deteriorating. The interior needed repainting, the linoleum on the kitchen floor needed replacing, the wall-to-wall carpet in one bedroom was splotched with wine and coffee stains. The improvised study where I did my writing and Natalyn worked on her slides was becoming hopelessly junked up.

What followed after we put down earnest money took up all our time and energy. It turned out that the new house had problems. A section of the foundation had a crack in it; there was water damage in the basement, carpenter bees had riddled the paint job, the clevis for the two-twenty house wire was loose. There were minor plumbing and electrical problems. The house was appraised at lower than its selling price. For over two months Natalyn and I dickered with the owner, trying to get her to lower the price. After obtaining minimal concessions from the owner, we had to come up with escrow money for the underwriters, and we didn't know whether our mortgage loan would be approved. On top of that, we had to find a renter for our old house, so Natalyn could keep the studio.

As it turned out, we found a renter in June, a graduate student in psychology, and our loan was finally approved. The closing took place on July 21. We gradually realized that, notwithstanding the crack in the foundation, the house had no serious structural damage, and once we had the eves cleaned out, we realized we would have no leakage problems.

I had kept Eileen up on our house problems, during my visits in April and May. When I had to postpone a visit, she seemed to understand. By this time she had another volunteer coming over, Lori Price, an Auburn University coed in pre-med. Sometimes the three of us were at Cassie's bedside. I could tell that Eileen wanted Lori, who was a little shy and very nice and proper, to feel comfortable. Eileen would talk to Lori while I drew a picture for Cassie. That's how it went with the three of us.

One afternoon late in May, Eileen and I were sitting in Eileen's bedroom. Lying in the hospital bed against one hall, Cassie was kneading her gums. The ceiling fan whickered, a pink and purple birthday balloon hovered over the metal footboard of the bed. Yes, it was Cassie's ninety-third birthday. She seemed aware of it; sometimes she eyed the drifting balloons. Warming up to Eileen's talk, a slight breeze filtering through the venetian blinds, I felt, for the time being at least, I belonged here. My life in Auburn seemed a long way off.

But once Natalyn and I began to settle into our new house, Eileen's house seemed increasingly remote. I was losing contact; I didn't want to call Eileen to make an appointment. Throughout August and early September, I found excuses for not going.

Another consequence of our moving into a new house was the suspension of this narrative. I didn't follow my usual practice of taking notes after each visit, usually at the Lazy Bee, a halfway point between Eileen's house and Auburn. Leaving Eileen's, I'd drive two miles to where Lee 27 deadended at Lee 54, take a right, and drive four or five miles to the Lazy Bee. I'd see sheep in a field to my right, a rusted-out harrow on my left, its crooked teeth a perpetual surprise, a lane to country houses for city folk, labeled SERENITY. I'd pass the millrace to my right, crossing the low plank bridge, knowing the Lazy Bee was just ahead. I'd pull into the parking lot near the picnic table—where, on one of my trips out, I'd wolfed down takeout fried chicken—and get out my black bound sketchbook. Without getting out of the car or even unhooking my seat belt, I'd jot the date down on a blank page. Then I'd scribble out notes, sketch cartoonish images of Eileen,

Cassie, Uncle Tim, James, myself, the living room, the bedroom. I would try to get down as much as I could remember in fifteen or twenty minutes.

A day or two later, I'd write a draft, converting my notes into narrative while each visit was still fresh in my mind. Sitting in a back booth at Burger King, I would write first drafts, usually early in the afternoon, for two or three hours at a sitting. Then I'd rewrite for two hours more, at home, on our Mac Performa. But once the process of buying a house was underway, I stopped the writing process. My notes lay unread in the black-bound sketchbook, from March to December.

Early in January 2000, over two months after Cassie died, I sat down at Burger King, had a Whopper Jr. with cheese for lunch, read the sports page of the *O-A News*, cleaned up the mess, got out a pen, a white legal pad, a cellophane bag of candy, and, finally, pulled the black-bound sketchbook out of the shoulder bag I had toted in from my car. I flipped through the entries, noted down the dates. I realized I could at least transcribe what I had, and perhaps in the process recover something of what I had felt. Some of the entries would be fragmentary; others I might be able to flesh out. I felt I had to try to get something down. What I did get down, perhaps it will speak for itself.

MARCH 11, 1999. While Eileen and I were with Cassie, a Hospice nurse showed up. She took Cassie's blood pressure, applied a stethoscope to Cassie's chest. A plump woman in her late thirties, frizzy, carrot-colored hair. She told us her husband had cut meat at Kroger's, from age seventeen on. "It could be our turn," she said to us. "We never know, someday someone will be looking after us."

A note on a sketch I did of Cassie. "She's smiling. She likes the drawing." Cassie looked at the sketch, turned it upside down and continued to peruse it. That could have been before or after the nurse came.

Eileen must have asked me to go to the living room while the nurse took Cassie's temperature, for on the next page, still dated March 11, are notes concerning a conversation I had with Eileen's son, James. I sketched him sitting across from me, noting that he was wearing a maroon jogging jacket and pants, contoured green sunglasses. I remember asking him about the trophies on the corner table, below his photograph and his sister's photograph. He took pleasure filling me in.

He'd won two trophies for most valuable player at Beauregard High School, another for most steals in one season. While he was in the Navy, stationed at Jacksonville, Florida, he was on a championship team participating in regional competition. He told me he had a scholarship offer from Amiville Junior College in Texas—that was before he joined the Navy, before he had the bone marrow transplant in Seattle. He said he'd wanted to go, but "Mama didn't want me to." He could have transferred from Beauregard High to a high school in Atlanta—he was that good—where he would have gotten more exposure. "It's done all the time, it's just something you never hear much about." But his mama didn't want him to leave home.

While we were in the living room, Eileen's Uncle Tim shuffled in from the kitchen. He sat down in Eileen's armchair, beaming at James as James went on about playing basketball. I have to say I was pleased to have a basketball player give me the time of day. I even tried to convey the impression that I knew the game fairly well. Since we were falling into the roles of two guys talking about sports, one old white guy, mostly listening, one young, but ailing, black guy talking, I thought I might slip in that I was once on the Vanderbilt fencing team. I think I told James I wasn't much of a basketball player, but I had done some fencing. It was clear from the perfunctory way James raised his eyebrows that he wasn't at all impressed.

MARCH 18. Cassie working her mouth, keeping her lips closed. I ask Eileen if Cassie ever took snuff. She took snuff once but she never smoked. No 'bacca, Eileen told me.

I have a sketch of us sitting on Eileen's double bed. I'm sitting next to the window. Usually Eileen sits next to the window.

Eileen must have gone out to do something, turn the oven down, put potatoes on to boil, giving me the opportunity to sketch her vanity. Radio, body lotions, hydrogen peroxide, Benedryl, petroleum jelly, a can of baby powder, ready-to-use throwaway enema bottles, more items than I can list.

There are two gargantuan safety pins pinned to the curtains in the bedroom window.

A black woman I haven't seen before comes in. Eileen regales this woman with her "Tale of the Erring Preacher." He preached at her church, Community of Jesus of the Apostolic Faith.

Here's what the erring preacher said to antagonize the older members of the congregation: "Old people ain't got no sense. They're all stooped over. They can't walk or run."

The erring preacher had been stealing money out of the collection plates. One time he tried to draw money out of the church bank account. The teller (white) told the preacher to leave or "we'll have the po-lice here."

Here is the erring preacher's last sermon. A stranger enters the church. The stranger sits down in one of the front pews. A little boy wants to touch the stranger's polished wingtips. His mama gives him a no-no. The stranger gets up out of the pew and strides out of the church. The po-lice are waiting for the erring preacher to finish up and leave the church. Two patrol cars, one in front, one in back, escort the erring preacher's car across the county line.

The erring preacher has a church in another county now. Since the erring preacher's departure, many young people have left the church. They've started going to the erring preacher's church in Opelika. Something is amiss here. Opelika is the county seat of Lee County, the county Eileen and I live in. But it is possible that the Community of Jesus is located in Macon County. The Macon County line is not that far from Eileen's house.

The stranger who mysteriously walked out of the church, who was he? The erring preacher's nemesis? Or a friend who wanted to warn him that the po-lice were waiting outside the church?

Actually, before returning to Auburn one afternoon, I drove the other way on Lee County 27, not toward Lee County 54 and the Lazy Bee. I wanted to have a look at the Community Church of Jesus, which, Eileen had informed me, should be just down the road. Two or three miles down this dismal road, nothing but pines and Keep Out signs lashed to barbed wire gates, I came upon this little white church with a hip roof and a minuscule steeple. I could have turned right at this church, taken another county road not far away, driven past an auto graveyard, veered off toward Beauregard Community, where Eileen's son James had once played basketball, passing the Beauregard Community fire station, clumps of houses, trailers, winding up somewhere south of Opelika. Or I could have gotten lost in a network of county roads. What I did after I passed the church was turn left, not right, doubling back to Lee County 54 via Lee County 47. I turned right on Lee County 54, passed the sheep, the harrow, the lane proclaiming SERENITY, returning to the Lazy Bee, parking, getting out my sketchbook. As for the church, it was a country church, but was it Eileen's church?

APRIL 1. In Auburn and Opelika, the azaleas are blossoming, redbuds, dogwoods, apple trees, forsythia. In Opelika signs with little red arrows are in place, designating what is known as the azalea trail leading through upper-middle-class residential areas. Along Lee County 54, there are patches of wisteria, sprinklings of dogwood, not much else.

A sports-utility van is parked in Eileen's front yard. I park behind it. Eileen opens the front door, and, stationing herself on the front steps, she motions for me to move my car. I park in the grass, well away from the sports-utility van parked in the driveway. The van, Eileen tells me, once I am in the living room, belongs to her new volunteer, Lori Price.

I have a sketch of the three of us sitting on Eileen's bed. I'm near the door, Lori is sitting next to me, Eileen is sitting by the window. Lori is wearing a white T-shirt, red lipstick flaking her thin lips. Lori brings up going to Australia this summer. She is really looking forward to it.

Cassie doesn't say much. She peruses my Easter egg sketch, done in colored pencils, which I'd brought along so I could do the sketch while I was there. I leave early, realizing Eileen would like to spend more time with Lori.

APRIL 15. I chat with Eileen in her living room. I'm in the rocker, she's in the armchair. Uncle Tim shuffles in from the hall leading to the bedrooms, a tobacco pouch protruding from his hip pocket. He moves on into the kitchen. Tim wants fresh catfish for dinner tonight, Eileen tells me. Where is he going to catch any catfish, Eileen says, he's too old to fish. Tim leaves the burner on in his trailer a lot. Eileen's afraid he will burn himself up. She has to do something about Tim. Maybe her doctor, Dr. Sibley, can get him in a nursing home, in Tuskegee, on his Medicaid.

Eileen tells me Cassie's been talking to dead people.

I'm alone with Cassie for awhile. She's been spitting up mucus, and since Eileen has to take the wash off the line, I'm the one who holds a shallow plastic basin up to Cassie's lips. She doesn't spit or drool in the basin, but her lips are damp so I wipe her lips off with Kleenex. The second time I hold up the bowl, Cassie takes it, birdclaw-like, then pushes it away. I wipe her lips with Kleenex, crumple a saliva-wet tissue, do a wastebasket drop. I have a note on this—"what does someone else's saliva feel like?"

Cassie is holding another sketch; her fingernails are a pale pink. In profile, her face, I'm thinking, resembles the American Indian head nickel. No, it doesn't, so why did that image pop into my head?

Returning, Eileen tells me her cousin braids Cassie's hair.

Dr. Sibley's mother, Mary Sibley, comes into Eileen's discourse. Eileen tells me Mary is the daughter of old Mrs. Sibley, whose husband sold Eileen's daddy the land for their house, a good bit of land, eighteen or so acres. Old Mrs. Sibley is in a nursing home. Cassie's sister helped raise Mary Sibley's children before Mary moved to Birmingham.

From time to time, Mary drives down from Birmingham to visit. She had a stroke that paralyzed three fingers, that has made driving a car difficult for her. Mary has to use these paralyzed three fingers of her left hand to steer so she can shift gears with her right hand, so she drives the back roads from Birmingham. Eileen sees Mary's driving as quite an accomplishment, and I agree, it most certainly is. On her visits, Mary sees her kinfolks; she stays at the Sibley house down the road. She'll stop over to visit Eileen. She gives Eileen money, which, Eileen says, she feels she can accept, for her aunt took care of Mary's children for years.

APRIL 29. Solid gray sky, off and on drizzle. Cassie's mind is wandering. With importunity, she utters the name of her dead sister, Susie Mae, she wants Susie Mae to do something for her. Weed the garden, yes. Cassie wants to be cooking something. She always liked to cook, but when her mind went, Eileen has told me more than once, Cassie stayed in the kitchen all the time. Cassie says she wants to pick blackberries with Justine. Who's Justine, I wonder. "You know you can't pick blackberries, sug," Eileen says firmly.

I'm thinking Cassie may know something we don't know. I remember what Bill Wanamaker told me over a beer at Touchdown's. Concerning the dying. "They know something we don't know."

I speculate on thought processes. Is Cassie's mind like stagnant water, a few thoughts drifting aimlessly? Or do her thoughts center on images that have a special meaning for her, picking blackberries with Justine, chopping cotton, her sister Susie Mae, her father, her mother, Eileen, James?

Later on we sit in the living room. I have a sketch—Eileen is wearing a broad striped shirt, a man's black hat, ankle length maroon slacks, white socks, pink slippers, the notes to my sketch tell me. She rubs her thighs as she talks to me. She twiddles her thumbs. I lean forward in the rocker, shift my legs.

Eileen is talking about diabetes. She calls it "the sugar." Her grandmother, her cousins, her father all had it, and she has it too, has had it for years. But she has kept it under control. After Eileen was diagnosed as diabetic, she was able to convince the nurse at EAMC that she could do her own insulin shots. She had given insulin shots to her grandmother and two of her cousins at the age of twelve. Her father had to have both legs amputated due to the sugar. He had to go to the hospital three times a week for dialysis. "They cut him in both arms. Then inside here." Eileen pats the inside of her thighs. "They were looking for a vein, for the dialysis. I don't know how he stood it." She wipes away a tear. "He worked so hard for us."

I am moved by her distress. "Your father must have been a strong man," I say, "and a good man."

May 20. Preoccupied with buying a house, I put off seeing Eileen for three weeks. My notes have dwindled down to incidental observations. "Window open half a foot. Black mesh of screen. Slight stirring of air in the room. Cassie's tight braids."

June 3. "Soap opera on in the living room. Gardenia, this from our old house, a present for Cassie. Trees not stirring outside the window."

June 11. "No change in Cassie. Ugly rent in wall paper, why doesn't Eileen have it patched up? At least tear off the dangling excrescence."

For the first time, I witness Eileen draining mucus from Cassie's throat. With her right hand, Eileen works the tube into Cassie's mouth, pushing it into her throat. With her left hand firmly pressing Cassie's nose, Eileen holds Cassie's head down.

Eileen reminisces on her childhood. She and her girls friends would go to a country store after school, before they went home and were put to work. They would pool their nickels to buy candy.

August 31. At the front door, I hear Eileen humming something sweet and spiritual. I'm surprised by what she is wearing, a sleeveless, low-cut, flowered dress.

We don't sit long in the living room. Eileen tells me Cassie is sleeping a lot, but she isn't in any pain. We go back to the bedroom. Eileen tells Cassie, "Mister Ross is here, sug" She means Mister Rose. Cassie's eyes are open, but she doesn't respond.

Eileen does most of the talking, on her favorite subject, what's wrong with how kids are raised today. "You don't tell a child you'll whip him next time. You do it right then and there." I bring up an instance of corporal punishment from my own childhood, my mother taking after my brother and myself with the flyswatter when we got out of hand. I don't say we used to sass and harass a young black woman, Ethel Lee (Ethel Lee was our maid for awhile), that when my mother had too much of this she went for the flyswatter.

It isn't long before we leave the bedroom. "Mister Ross is leaving, sug," Eileen says to Cassie. Cassie comes out of her torpor and says, "thank you."

I don't leave the house right way, sensing Eileen wants to talk some more. She's back in the armchair, in the living room, and I'm asking her how James is doing. James has been in Atlanta, she tells me, for several weeks. He's been working with a friend on this rich white woman's house. They're putting in ceiling fans, rewiring, Eileen doesn't specify what else. The pay is good, and James gets all he wants to eat. Eileen expatiates on the opulence she's heard about from James—clothes closets the size of two rooms, Maine lobster flown in, a chauffeured limo. James comes home on weekends. He returns to her house, to his tiny corner bedroom across from Eileen and Cassie's bedroom. He's been living in Eileen's house for the last several years.

We talk some more. Eileen lambastes the internet, claiming it has a pernicious impact on young people. Eileen had read something very disturbing concerning the internet in the *O-A News*. Right down the road, at Beauregard High School, a fourteen-year-old black girl contacted two men from New York City on the internet. It was arranged for them to drive down from New York. They would pick this girl up in front of the high school. One day she got off the school bus and got into a car with New York license plates. Several weeks later the girl called her parents, and her mother went to New York and brought the girl back. Her mother put the New York police onto the culprits, who were arrested, who, Eileen is hoping, will do time. Prisons, she says, are too soft anymore. Hardened criminals just sit around and watch

TV. "I'd have them on the road gangs, the way it used to be."

An hour and a half later I say I have to be going. I say, "Next time I won't take so long getting here."

Eileen says, "I've missed seeing you. I know I talk all the time."

I look down at the pea green porcelain cats stored under the coffee table, then back at Eileen. So she talks a lot; she needs to talk. "I've enjoyed seeing you," I say. "It's been nice coming out here."

Eileen unlocks the screen door and lets me out. A black man I haven't seen before is mowing the lawn, cutting broad swathes with a riding lawn mower. He smiles, waves at us. Uncle Tim is sitting out back beside the butane tank.

At the Lazy Bee I take a close look at the bee rebus. I sketch it out again because I didn't get it right the first time. I'm being a stickler for verisimilitude. I get down a pretty good likeness of a cartoonish bumblebee shaped like a peanut—black-striped yellow body, white wings, incongruous tan sneakers. What were the sneakers all about? The red tongue hanging out of a yum yum grin, why hadn't I noticed that tongue before?

Another note, on August 31, concerning my stopover at the Lazy Bee. This one, possibly, showing synchronicity. "Bee inside car window?" Inside my car, windows closed? In that case turn the engine on, lower the window so the bee—a honeybee? a wasp?—can find a way out before I get stung.

SEPTEMBER 16. Eileen has gone to the kitchen. She has butterbeans simmering on the stove and needs to check on them. After she comes back, I feel some tension between us. Eileen is off on the drugs, the killings, raising children again. To get her off this, I ask about James. He's still in Atlanta, she says curtly. Abruptly, she asks, "Shall we go see Cassie?"

The tension goes with us to the bedroom, so right away I do a drawing of Cassie. I show it to Eileen and, as usual, she thanks me, and says to Cassie, "It looks just like you, sug." She hands the drawing back to me. It goes easier between us now. I'm guiding Cassie's hands around the drawing, on a page of notebook paper. Cassie looks at it, uttering a barely audible "thank you." She turns it upside down, continues to hold on to it.

Pretty soon I'm telling Eileen about taking high school art, back in Kokomo High School. I used to think I might be an artist, but I never learned to use oils or watercolors, and my perspective was awry. My high school art teacher (an eccentric spinster who lived in the Courtland Hotel on North Main Street) used to tell me, "Charles, you can draw a pretty good likeness, but you don't know how to put the shadows in." Eileen listens with interest. I tell her my high school art teacher was right, I wasn't meant to be an artist. One of my high school English teachers encouraged me to write, and while I wouldn't call myself a writer, I've published stories and done some writing. Eileen tells me, "Sometimes things don't turn out the way we expect them to."

Again we're taking pleasure in talking to each other. The conversation meanders to Eileen's job, in housekeeping at East Alabama Medical Center, known as Lee County hospital while she was working there. She tells me the floors had to be mopped right. After mopping three or four rooms, she had to change the water. She had to change the mop heads every two hours. What we are talking about isn't that important, what *is* is that we are talking.

After awhile, Eileen goes to the kitchen to check on the butterbeans, leaving me alone with Cassie. Mid-afternoon sunlight is gilding the bedrail. Cassie is working her mouth, kneading her gums, one knobby knee puffing the thin cotton blanket. There's a bubble of drool on her lips. I move the basin up under her lips.

This time she pushes it away. I wipe her lips off with Kleenex. A butterbean aroma drifts in from the kitchen. Gazing out through the venetian blinds at the front yard, I let my eyes rest on the fire hydrant next to the road.

SEPTEMBER 23. The nights are getting chilly, but we're having another warm afternoon in September, in the low eighties.

Eileen wears a baggy, striped dress, a large safety pin showing in the tight cloth below her breasts. We're in the living room. She tells me right away—she and James have put Tim in a nursing home in Tuskegee. Doctor Sibley has arranged for Medicaid to pay for it. Tim had complained a lot about having to go to a nursing home, and she'd been afraid they would have to make him go. But as the time drew near, he changed his mind. She bought new clothes for him, a bathrobe, and a pair of new shoes, which he had insisted on putting on that day. After that, Tim couldn't wait to go.

Eileen tells me she was impressed with how clean the nursing home looked. She makes a point of emphasizing that the people at the nursing home, both black folks and white folks, seemed to get along well.

We go back to see Cassie. I do another drawing of her, for her. She turns it upside down. She holds it for awhile.

OCTOBER 21. For nearly a month I had put off scheduling another visit. When I did call Eileen, on the morning of the twenty-first, I got a busy signal. That afternoon I ran some errands; then, settled into the back booth of Burger King, I did some work on a short story. When I got back home, around five, Natalyn told me there was a message from Linda Merritt on the answering machine. The message was brief—Cassie Binton had passed away late Wednesday night. Natalyn and I talked about Cassie Binton for awhile.

She suggested I call Eileen, if not tonight, then early tomorrow. I would have to wait until tomorrow to call Linda Merritt.

I didn't call Eileen that night. There was another message on the answering machine, from Amy Willis, my doubles partner in the Auburn Tennis League's Thursday night competitions. One of the men on our team couldn't make it tonight. If I couldn't get there myself, I should let Amy know immediately. I called Amy Willis and said I would be there. I would put off calling Eileen until tomorrow.

Under the lights, with people I didn't know well, tennis enthusiasts rated from 2.5 to 3.5, memories of Eileen's bedroom, Cassie lying in the hospital bed surfaced unexpectedly, while I was changing courts, zipping up my racket bag after the matches were over. On the way home, I picked up Woody Allen's "Wild Man Blues" at Blockbusters, $3.99 for a five-day rental. I wouldn't be watching Woody Allen play New Orleans jazz, not tonight, tomorrow, or the next day. By the time I got back to the house, my legs were stiff and sore from tendonitis.

We had lentil soup for supper that night. We ate the soup in front of the television set, watched "Law and Order," the ten o'clock Alabama news, then Jay Leno. Natalyn went on to bed. I stayed up reading Harold Bloom on Shakespeare's "King John" and "Henry VI." I was expecting it to turn cold, so I set the thermostat at sixty-five; then I hobbled to the bathroom and took a hot bath. I took two Tylenol PM's for the tendonitis and flopped down beside Natalyn. It wasn't long before I was asleep.

At four AM I awoke to what sounded like a branch scratching against the window. Natalyn was still asleep. I realized that the scratching was due to a malfunction in the electric alarm clock. As I was on the point of drifting back to sleep, the scratching persisting, Cassie's image blended with that of my own grandmother. I remembered how it was for my grandmother Beck, nearly twenty-five year ago. She was lying in another hospital bed, in a nursing home on the western boundary of Kokomo. My mother was nagging at her to take out her false teeth; my mother insisted on cleaning them. My grandmother kept her lips tightly closed. "Are you listening to me, Mother. I want you to take out your false teeth." Mother Beck, my father used to call her. My grandmother Beck finally opened her mouth. She gave up. My mother removed the false teeth. Grandmother Beck, ninety-one now, past propriety, forgetting her corseted, querulous pleasure-denying ways, gazed at me as if I were a desirable male, asking my mother "who's your beau, is that nice looking man your beau?" My mother hastened to tell her, "that's Charles, that's your grandson, Charles."

I thought of my mother, Josephine Beck Rose—she had not withered away in a hospital bed, she had died suddenly, six hundred miles away from me, in a hospital in Kokomo. She was eighty-seven. Just a week after I visited her in Kokomo she called me from the hospital. She had had persistent diarrhea for several weeks. During my visit I had urged her to go to the hospital, but I hadn't taken her myself. The night before I drove back to Auburn, I watched her measuring out olive juice for our martinis. I remembered descending the creaking stairs—I slept in one of the rooms upstairs in the same bed I'd slept in as a child, with the window open—tiptoeing into the cluttered downstairs bathroom to pee, hearing my mother stir fitfully in her bedroom. I remembered her false teeth soaking in a milky jelly glass.

The alarm clock kept on scratching. A line from Wallace Stevens came to me, from "Peter Quince at the Clavier."

> Susannah's music touched the bawdy strings
> Of those white elders, but, escaping,
> Left only death's ironic scraping.

Those ladies, my grandmother, my mother, long departed, where had they gone?

OCTOBER 22. Late on Friday morning I left a message with Linda Merritt. Then I touched-toned Eileen's number. I was relieved when James answered, for I didn't know what to say to Eileen.

"Hello," I said briskly. "Is this James?"

"Hey there." I could tell James recognized my voice. His own was friendly, reassuring.

"It's me. Charles Rose, Cassie's Hospice volunteer. My director, Linda Merritt, called me to tell me Cassie had passed away. I'm so sorry to hear that." Something like that.

I don't remember what James said next. Or did I keep on talking? "Could you tell me about the funeral arrangements?"

"The funeral is this Sunday, at two PM. It's at Community of Jesus Church. That's right down the road from where we live."

I remembered the white frame church I had seen several weeks ago, its hip roof, its minuscule steeple. "Yes, I know where that is." And then, "Would you tell Eileen I'll be there for the funeral? And please give her my condolences?"

"I'll do that."

I don't remember how the phone call ended. I did ask James to tell me the name of the church again. He told me it was the Community of Jesus of the Apostolic Faith.

"Sense of a burden lifted," my black-bound sketchbook reads. "Relief, tranquility."

OCTOBER 24. Now comes a comedy of errors, my errors.

Sunday morning, the day of the funeral. I took my time dressing. I put on gray pants, a white shirt, black shoes and socks, a subdued maroon regimental tie, a navy blue blazer. Over a late breakfast, Natalyn and I talked about the funeral, what it might be like. I left the house at 1:20 P.M., estimating that it would take me twenty minutes to half an hour to get to the church, with ten minutes to spare before the service commenced. Another sunny October day. On Lee 27, I saw a cluster of cars parked outside of Eileen's house. For a second or two, I thought of stopping to confirm James's directions, but that would take time, and, most likely, nobody would be there during the funeral.

Again the desolate, pine-hedged road opened out ahead. Near the end of Lee 27, I reached the white frame church with the minuscule steeple. Instead of people entering the church, they were *coming out*, black couples, children, all in their Sunday best, clustering, chatting outside the church before getting into their washed and waxed automobiles and, yes, *driving away*. I pulled into the parking lot. Two soberly attired black men approached me, no doubt deacons. They stood by the car, waiting for me to roll down the window on the driver's side and explain what I was doing there. I needed to get the window down, talk to them, even though the sign in front of the church said Bethel Baptist Church instead of Community of Jesus Church of the Apostolic Faith. In my confusion and dismay, I pressed the wrong switch. Water squirted onto my windshield. One of the deacons couldn't conceal a smirk; the other kept a straight face. I found the right switch, the front window glided down. Then I asked the deacons if they could tell me how to find Community of Jesus Church. One said he didn't know; the other, trying to help, launched into elaborate directions I knew I couldn't follow. Take a right at the junkyard on Lee 47, keep on going to Lee 51, on through Beauregard, take a right, a left. I thanked both deacons and backed out of the parking lot. I might still get to the funeral.

I took Lee 47 to the auto graveyard, sunlight pounding down on rusted metal. I turned right, and, arriving at Lee 51, I recognized a church I had been in before. It was the Methodist church where Howard Carr's funeral had been held, over a year ago. I backtracked to Bethel Baptist, now deserted, and on past Eileen's house. Cars were still clustered in the front yard, so the funeral must be going on somewhere. Reaching Lee 54, I took a left instead of a right, thinking Community of Jesus might be in Macon County. After crossing the Macon County line, I remembered that James had told me the church was right down the road. He must have meant the road Eileen lived on. So I gave up. Cassie's funeral would soon be over. I quickly rejected the option of showing up at Eileen's house after the funeral. By 3 P.M. I was back in Auburn. I bought a condolence card at the nearest drug store.

I called Eileen later on that afternoon. A young girl answered the telephone.

"Could I talk to Eileen Foote?"

"I'll get her."

In Eileen's crowded living room, a hubbub of clamorous black folks, male and female. Then Eileen was on the telephone. I apologized right off; I said I must have gotten James's directions wrong. She told me quickly where the church was located. My error had been simple. Community of Jesus wasn't on Lee 27 at all; it was somewhere on a narrow, unmarked road veering off from Lee 27, to the right, she told me. I must have passed it without seeing its tunnel-like opening into dense pine, just before Lee 27 hooked up with Bethel Baptist.

I said to Eileen, "Now I realize why I couldn't find it." Eileen must have said something over the hubbub. "I know it was a lovely service," I blurted out, and then, "I know it's good to have your family with you."

"Yes it is," Eileen said. There was a pause.

"I'll call you later on in the week, if that's okay."

"That will be fine. Thank you," she said.

As soon as I was off the line I felt an assuagement of guilt. At least I had talked to her.

October 25. On Monday, I telephoned Linda Merritt at her office, and told her I'd missed the funeral. "That's too bad," she said, "but sometimes these mix-ups happen." She went on to say, "Maybe you should wait awhile, say a week or two, before you see her again. That is when she may really need to see you."

November 7. I'm sitting in an armchair in Eileen's living room. She has two visitors, in addition to myself. Sitting across from me on the sofa is Ella. Ella is a small, reserved woman with frizzy gray hair, wearing a turquoise beret, a dark blue, long-sleeved polka dot blouse. She has a paper cup in one hand, its straw protruding. She fiddles with the straw with her other hand while she listens to her sister, Wilhamena, hold forth in the rocker, on the other side of a rubber plant to my left. Wilhamena is a tall, vociferous woman, her chin jutting out, spectacles riding her nose.

Eileen is ensconced in her armchair. She is wearing maroon slacks and pink slippers, a green pullover sweater. The ceramic cats are still stationed under the coffee table. On the shelf attached over the sofa, the ceramic dogs, the elephant, the white rooster with glassy red crest keep a deferential quietude. A gift for Eileen, wrapped and ribboned, something Natalyn picked up for Eileen at Big Lots, remains where I put it when I arrived, on the table next to Eileen's armchair. I hear other visitors confabulating in the kitchen.

The women are Eileen's cousins. Ella, the timid, polka-dotted cousin, I've been informed by Eileen at the door, has had a stroke. Her voice pipes up infrequently in a faint antiphonal response, an "ain't that the truth" or "oh yes" to Wilhamena's frequent vociferations. Soon we are talking about Cassie (I have expressed my condolences and Eileen has accepted them graciously). Eileen tells us what a good woman Cassie was. She talks about the garden Cassie kept, what a good cook she was, how much she loved her sister, Susie Mae.

Wilhamena brings up Cassie's other sister, Mattie Elizabeth. Mattie Elizabeth, Wilhamena informs us, got tired of being called Mattie Elizabeth, but Cassie, she just wouldn't stop using Mattie Elizabeth's middle name because she knew that was the right thing to do. Pretty soon, I bring up what Cassie said when I showed her the first drawing I did of her. "Well I declare," I say. We all smile and chuckle over this. The women continue to talk about Cassie. From the kitchen, other voices.

The talk gets around to James's new job in Atlanta. Eileen expatiates on the thirteen-room mansion with dressing rooms "as large as this room," all the fine clothes this rich woman has, "so much good food." The chauffeur, she says with awe, makes eight hundred dollars a week. From Wilhamena, strong appreciation, from Ella, "oh yes." There is a lull in the conversation. I'm wondering if I should ask Eileen if she would like to open her gift. No, she would rather wait until the cousins leave. Which they do, after what seems like a long decent interval. Wilhamena gets up first, towering over the potted palm. She goes to Ella and helps her up from the sofa. Soon they are at the front door, on their way.

I ask Eileen if she would like to open her gift. She says she would. Reaching over to the end table she picks up the package, peels off the tissue and ribbons.

She holds up a plastic cylinder with a lid on it, containing dried flower petals, many hued, spicy. She gives me a big smile and says, "Well, isn't that nice."

"You can pour it out in a saucer, or around a candle, my wife tells me, so it will scent the air. She thought you might like it."

"Thank your wife for me." And then, movingly, "Bless her."

I say, "I know Natalyn will appreciate your saying that."

We sit quietly for awhile. The talk in the kitchen is dying down. I've never seen Eileen look so despondent. I ask her how she's feeling, and she tells me she isn't sleeping much. She hasn't been able to sleep since Cassie passed.

"I'm tired all the time, but once I lie down on the bed I know I'll never get to sleep."

I'm trying to be helpful, in any way I can. "I know it isn't easy for you. You've had to take on so much responsibility."

"Yes, I was taking care of Cassie; that took up most of my time. Now I don't know what to do with myself."

Eileen tugs at the sleeves of her sweater. I say, "That's natural. You've been through a lot, and now it's over."

"I know, I know. And there's a lot to be done, but I can't make myself do anything." She folds her hands, looks up. "Jesus will show me the way. He always has, and He will now."

"Yes," I say, "that's right."

"I am going to rake the leaves though. The front yard really needs it."

"That sounds like a good idea," I say. I ask Eileen if she's been back to her church, and she says, "Yes, last Sunday. The people there, they remember me."

"After all the time you were unable to go, it's good that they remember you. And since you've been having trouble sleeping, you might take something at night. I'm not talking about sleeping pills. You could take something like Tylenol PM to relax you. That's what I do at night and it helps me sleep."

"Yes, I'll get some. Maybe that will help."

Coming in from the kitchen, a loose-limbed young black woman replaces the cordless receiver on the wall cradle in the hall. Without looking at us, she returns to the kitchen. The seconds trickle on. We've been sitting here much as we used to, only this time we won't go back to see Cassie. I know I shouldn't go to that bedroom again; yet something makes me want to have a last look at it.

"Wilhamena and me, we did clean Tim's trailer. It was a sight. I thank the Lord I was able to get Tim into a nursing home.'

I look up at the drawing I did of the house, on the wall across the living room. Tim's trailer is poking out from one side of the house, on the side where Eileen's bedroom is. Blue skies over the house, swollen cumuli over the pines. "You were telling me Tim likes the nursing home."

"He didn't want to go for so long, but when the time came he couldn't wait to go." I'm hearing, with relief, her story of how Tim got to the nursing home. Eileen knows I've heard the story before, but she goes on; why not? The time passes quickly now.

She tells stories, or pieces of stories. About James's bone marrow transplant in Seattle, about growing up, how hard she had to work as a girl, cooking, cleaning, watering the hogs, chopping cotton. How she looked after her father when he got the sugar. Her father stayed in the room James was living in now, the room her father and mother kept her grandfather in; that was after she was married and living with her husband in Tuskegee. "We did for each other," Eileen says, "Most families don't do that anymore."

I tell her a story concerning my own family. It goes back almost sixty years. It's about Granny Rose, my father's mother. She was a perky woman with cottony white hair. She was in her seventies, bedridden most of the time, due to her arthritis. She could only get around with a walking cane. Eileen is listening; that I am aware of as I spin out the story of Granny Rose.

Granny Rose spent the winter months with my Uncle Kenneth and Aunt Hazel in Nashville, Tennessee. During the spring and summer she lived with us, in Kokomo. Twice a year, Granny Rose (her given name was Jesse Rose) would get in one of her sons' automobiles, either in Nashville or in Kokomo, and, with either Uncle Kenneth or my father doing the driving, go to a halfway meeting point, in Louisville, Kentucky.

There she would change automobiles and sons, proceeding, with my father or Uncle Kenneth, either to Kokomo or Nashville. I can remember seeing my father help Granny get out of his Buick, the good feeling I had seeing him back with Granny. My father would escort Granny through the back porch and kitchen of our two-story Victorian house, through the living room, down the hall to the back bedroom, *her* bedroom.

Granny would get into her double bed, and, as soon as she was settled, she would turn on the Philco radio on her bedside table. She would get WGN in Chicago. The next day—it must have been a Sunday, for it had to be on a Saturday that Granny's homecoming took place—my brother, Richard, and I would spend the afternoon in Granny's room. I don't remember how old we were then. I might have been anywhere from seven to nine, my brother six to eight. The three of us would listen to the Cubs game on WGN. Our bird dog, Spot, would scramble up onto Granny's double bed. Granny lay beside the window, the Philco sharing her bedtable with an electric fan and various medicines we never identified.

Granny Rose was an ardent Cub fan. A victory for the Cubs would make her day. Even splitting a doubleheader was good. As the years wore on for her, there were all too many days of defeat for the three of us to get over.

Granny Rose died in Nashville, away from us. She was buried in Nashville, not Kokomo.

After an hour and a half of story telling, Eileen is yawning and I am getting restless and hungry. I ask her what she's going to do over Thanksgiving. She'll spend Thanksgiving with James and her daughter, at her daughter's place in Atlanta. If she feels up to it. Before I leave, she asks me to thank my wife for the gift. "I hope you can bring your wife with you sometime."

"I'll try to do that," I reply tentatively, for I'm not sure Natalyn would want to come with me. And I might not be coming back myself.

Other voices, from the kitchen. Eileen walks me to the door.

"I'll see you next Tuesday. Or next Thursday," I say, once I'm outside. Eileen is standing behind the closed screen door.

"Make it Thursday, if that is convenient," she says.

"All right, Thursday. I'll call you before I come," I say.

NOVEMBER 18. Pulling into the driveway, I see that the leaves have been raked up in the front yard. Eileen's brother, Charles, is getting into his car. I haven't seen him for months, not since we sat in the living room, and he talked to me about retiring from Uniroyal. He waves a casual greeting, but that's it, he's on his way out. I'm facing the front door with its diagonally descending glass panels, the front window with its three curtains, the TV aerial next to the front door, the brick foundation. Beyond the scraggly pines, the sky is gray.

Soon I'm seated in the rocker. Eileen is sitting in the armchair. Today she is wearing a green sweater, dark blue sweat pants, black socks, tan perforated, open-toed shoes. No other visitors, just us. The space heater is on, its blue flames flickering. I've asked Eileen about her Thanksgiving plans. Will she be visiting her son and daughter in Atlanta? No, they will be visiting her. She'll probably spend Christmas with them. All this is said in a flat perfunctory way. I sense Eileen tightening up, withdrawing.

I have to ask her how she is taking Cassie's death.

She's sitting rigidly in the armchair, her shoulders hunched, her hands clenched. "Sut," she's calling Cassie Binton, Sut. "Sut's right arm and leg were stiff, and she was coughing. Her kidneys failed. I tried to get a little milk into her, but the milk, it wouldn't go down." She draws her shoulders in a little, her fingers locked, her eyes bulging.

I say, "You were using the feeding tube?"

"Yes, the tube, but it wouldn't go. It didn't do any good."

"Did she get enough morphine?"

"Yes, she did; I don't know how much pain she had, but the coughing, that didn't stop. And she was choking up from the mucus. I had to keep draining mucus out of her throat. I was up with her all the time, but it was no use. I knew Jesus was going to take her."

I'm leaning forward in the rocker, not knowing how I might appear to her because I'm fastening on every word she says, trying to find a way for her to get through Cassie's suffering.

Finally, I ask her, "What was Cassie like when she passed away?"

Eileen's body relaxes, her hands drift apart. Her face takes on serenity. "Sut died in her sleep. She went to sleep like a baby." Tears are beading her eyes, my eyes are moistening.

She says, "Jesus took her like a baby."

I haven't seen Eileen since I left that day. It was mid-December when I telephoned her. I'd brought a poinsettia for her, which was something I'd done the Christmas before. Now I asked her if I could bring it by.

"I'm not going to be here today," Eileen said, a purposeful firmness in her voice. "I appreciate your thoughtfulness. You give the poinsettia to your wife. I know she'll appreciate it."

"I'll do that," I said, and, after a pause, "I'll give you a call after Christmas.'

"That will be fine," she said, but we both knew I wouldn't be seeing her again.

Later that day, Natalyn and I talked about what had happened. It might not look right for me to continue visiting Eileen, for I was a white male. Perhaps her daughter told her this, or James might have, or her brother Charles, or people in her church. I had gotten hints of distrust before, but hints only, nothing explicit. Or Eileen might have her own reasons. Certainly, she must have realized that she had revealed a lot to me.

I did send Eileen a Christmas card, with a note. "Our best to you and your family."

IN JANUARY, Linda Merritt called to tell me she had a male patient for me. She told me he lived in Auburn. His wife needed someone to sit with him while she ran errands.

I asked Linda what the illness was. Linda told me the patient had a bronchial condition. She said she would accompany me on the first visit, as she had in the past. Or, if I preferred, she would give me the address, and I could go without her.

I asked her what the address was. It was 307 Bowden Drive. The patient's house was next door to the house we had left, the house we were currently renting out.

Ed Cronin had been our neighbor. He used to work at the post office; then he'd retired and bought the house next door. Neither of us were neighborly, although we were friendly when we happened to meet.

I remember taking a letter addressed to Ed Cronin out of my mailbox, crossing the property line to Ed's front walls. His house was much like ours, small, with asbestos shingling. It had a carport instead of a double garage. Ed's wife came to the door, and I gave her the letter. We chatted for a little while. I had no idea Ed was terminally ill.

A week went by, without my hearing anything more from Linda Merritt. I called her at her office, and she told me the patient's wife would rather have a woman to sit with her husband. I'm not sure that was Ed Cronin's only reason for not accepting me as a volunteer. Perhaps he didn't want a former neighbor to sit with him.

As I write this sentence, I'm not sure whether I'll go on being a Hospice volunteer. One thing is certain. A story has to stop somewhere. Mine, I say to myself, will stop here, with the author seated in a booth at Burger King, on a sunny winter day in February, windowed off from a cloudless wash of sky, from the all-too-familiar buildings of downtown Auburn.

Looking Back

E ARLY IN THE following year I realized I had osteoarthritis in both hips. No cartilage in either, bone spurs in the right hip. I would be using a cane for the next four years. Due to my infirmity, and to a reluctance to keep on doing what I'd done, I drifted away from Hospice.

I made one last visit as a volunteer. This time I went to Bethany House, Hospice's new facility for patients unable to be treated at home. There I met a new patient, Betsy Williams, a white woman, in her late fifties, maybe early sixties. She didn't have any family—the nurse had told me—to visit her. Yet in spite of that she was in good spirits. We carried on an animated conversation for over an hour, in her room at one end of a corridor, sunlight streaming through the Venetian blinds, shrubbery outside, an azure sky wisped with cirrus clouds. I remember her telling me she had been married twice. She loved to fish with her second husband. She told me they'd spent weekends in a cabin on the Chattahoochee River.

On the following Saturday, I went back to Bethany House. I was looking forward to seeing Betsy Williams again. At the nursing station I got some good news. One of the nurses told me Betsy had been sent home on Friday. My image of Betsy Williams in her hospital bed, chatting with me, has remained untarnished, scintillating with life.

So what does it all come down to? I have asked that question of myself many times. From the vantage point of illusory stasis, brought on by retirement and advancing age, I'm tempted be an optimist, seeing the future as a broad, open road leading on to something better. The fact is such optimism is really a form of self-protection.

A onetime reader of Franz Kafka, I can detect some similarity in my urge for self-protection to that of Kafka's prairie dog in "The Burrow": "I have completed the construction of my burrow," the story begins, "and it seems to be successful." Sometimes I think of myself as safely lodged in my burrow, sandbagged with avoidance mechanisms, pleasantly foolish distractions. This is especially easy when you have fewer commitments. My teaching career was over, my children were grown and doing fairly well.

Other times, I identify myself with Land Surveyor K. in The Castle. Up to a point, needless to say, for no mysterious bureaucracy is standing in my way. Nonetheless, the feeling has persisted—one keeps plodding on, unable to break out of existence, its multilayered contradictions, its crooked roads that seem to lead nowhere.

Another possibility for me at this stage of life inheres in Kafka's aphorism, from "Reflections on Sin, Pain, Hope, and the True Way": "Theoretically there exists a perfect possibility for happiness: to believe in the indestructible element in oneself and not strive after it." Theoretically. There's the catch. Even though I'm pretty sure I saw UFOs one night, lights anyway, flitting and dipping in the sky, I'm not one to believe in revelation with a capital R.

Yet there are times when, summoning memories of being a

Hospice volunteer, I sense a tremulous synchronicity in the look and feel of a room, an appreciative glance, shared silences, the play of sunlight, a leaf moving in the wind. These three men and this woman, Lonnie Simmons, Howard Carr, Larry Beckwith, Cassie Binton, in their last days they have borne home to me the incommensurable distance between this world and what lies beyond. And in memory they still have a face, a voice, as one might say of a departed loved one. Their caregivers, those close to them, Mary Wagner, Helen Carr, Katherine Beckwith, Eileen Foote, I can envision, even converse with them as they were when I was with them. I can say I was of some help to them, as I believe I was from time to time. Certainly, they were of help to me. But that was transitory, what we said and did. Beyond what I have gotten down in this book, there was a shimmering in the air evocative of something ineffable, tentative yet palpable, elusive yet real.

A little over four years have passed since Cassie Binton died. On an Easter Sunday, after attending a Unitarian service, Natalyn and I drove out to Eileen Foote's place. No sun, the sky looked forbidding. After making the wrong turn—onto Lee County Road 47, not Lee 27, I backtracked, drove on a mile or so on Lee 54, turned left onto Lee 27. It seemed to take forever to get to the house. Finally, at the bottom of a long grade, we came upon it, set back from the road, to our left. The house seemed much smaller than I remembered it, hudding behind the front yard, the clay driveway as if it didn't want to be seen from the road.

I passed the house without stopping. Half a mile or so down the road, I turned the car around, and we returned the way we had come. I took a descending ess curve, approaching the house. Natalyn had a digital camera with her, having taken photographs of the Lazy Bee, the millrace, sheep grazing in a pasture. Just this side of the pale green fire hydrant, I stopped the car. Natalyn got out with her camera. Skirting clumps of saw grass, clusters of prickly thistles on the roadside, she took a photograph of the fire hydrant, the stolid mailbox. The house, the wash house out back, the pines, the cottony sky memorialized the fleeting moment.

About the Author

CHARLES ROSE taught English at Auburn University for thirty-four years. A native of Indiana, he holds degrees from Vanderbilt and the University of Florida and has published many short stories and articles. This is his first book. He lives in Auburn, Alabama. He is a past Hospice Volunteer of the Year, and in 2004 he was awarded an Alabama State Council on the Arts Fellowship for literary arts/fiction.

www.ingramcontent.com/pod-product-compliance
Lightning Source LLC
Chambersburg PA
CBHW031511270326
41930CB00006B/359